Basic Mechanisms
of Digestive Diseases:
the Rationale
for Clinical Management
and Prevention

John Libbey Eurotext
127, avenue de la République
92120 Montrouge
Tél. : 33 (0) 1 46 73 06 60
e-mail : contact@john-libbey-eurotext.fr
http://www.john-libbey-eurotext.fr

John Libbey and Company Ltd
Collier House,
163-169 Brompton Road, Knightsbridge
London SW3 1 PY, England
Tel. : 44 (0) 20 75 81 24 49

© John Libbey Eurotext, 2002
ISBN : 2-7420-0439-4

Il est interdit de reproduire intégralement ou partiellement le présent ouvrage - loi du 11 mars 1957 - sans autorisation de l'éditeur ou du Centre Français du Copyright, 6 *bis*, rue Gabriel-Laumain, 75010 Paris.

Basic Mechanisms of Digestive Diseases: the Rationale for Clinical Management and Prevention

Edited by
M.J.G. Farthing
P. Malfertheiner

Postgraduate Course 2002
Geneva, October 20

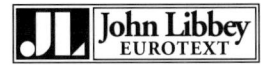

The publication of this book was made possible
thanks to the support from the NEGMA-GILD Laboratories.

Contents

List of contributors VII

Gastroesophageal reflux disease

New drug developments in gastroesophageal reflux disease
J.P. Galmiche 1

Advances in treatment strategies for gastroesophageal reflux disease
L. Lundell 13

Inflammatory bowel disease

New insights in the molecular etiopathogenesis of inflammatory bowel disease
J. Schölmerich 23

Drug development based on the molecular mechanisms and current strategies for therapy of inflammatory bowel disease
S. Schreiber 35

Irritable bowel syndrome

Irritable bowel syndrome and other functional bowel disorders. New answers to old questions
P. Enck, H. Hinninghofen 47

Irritable bowel syndrome: new drugs and therapeutic horizons
M.J.G. Farthing 59

Colon cancer

New approaches to management of gastrointestinal stromal tumors
F. Farinati, R. Cardin, M. De Giorgio, S. Gianni 75

Liver cancer

Basic mechanisms of liver cancer
H.E. Blum, D. Moradpour 83

Liver cancer. Multimodality approaches to treatment
*P. Schemmer, A. Mehrabi, P. Büchler, A.A. Tempia-Caliera, H. Friess,
M.W. Büchler* 97

Prevention of hepatocellular carcinoma
Th. Poynard, V. Ratziu 115

List of contributors

Blum H.E., Department of Medicine II, University of Freiburg, Hugstetter strasse 55, D-79106 Freiburg, Germany.

Büchler P., Department of General Surgery, Ruprecht-Karls, University of Heidelberg, Im Neuenheimer Feld 110 (Kirschnerstr. 1), D-69120 Heidelberg, Germany.

Büchler M.W., Department of General Surgery, Ruprecht-Karls, University of Heidelberg, Im Neuenheimer Feld 110 (Kirschnerstr. 1), D-69120 Heidelberg, Germany.

Cardin R., Section of Gastroenterology, Department of Surgical and Gastroenterological Sciences, via Giustiniani 2, 35128 Padua, Italy.

De Giorgio M., Section of Gastroenterology, Department of Surgical and Gastroenterological Sciences, via Giustiniani 2, 35128 Padua, Italy.

Enck P., University Hospitals Tübingen, Department of General Surgery, Waldhörnlestr. 22, 72072 Tübingen, Germany.

Farinati F., Section of Gastroenterology, Department of Surgical and Gastroenterological Sciences, via Giustiniani 2, 35128 Padua, Italy.

Farthing M.J.G., Faculty of Medicine, University of Glasgow, Glasgow G12 8LG, United Kingdom.

Friess H., Department of General Surgery, Ruprecht-Karls, University of Heidelberg, Im Neuenheimer Feld 110 (Kirschnerstr. 1), D-69120 Heidelberg, Germany.

Galmiche J.-P., Department of Gastroenterology and Hepatology and CIC-INSERM, Hôtel-Dieu, 44093 Nantes Cedex, France.

Gianni S., Section of Gastroenterology, Department of Surgical and Gastroenterological Sciences, via Giustiniani 2, 35128 Padua, Italy.

Hinninghofen H., University Hospitals Tübingen, Department of General Surgery, Waldhörnlestr. 22, 72072 Tübingen, Germany.

Lundell L., Department of Surgery, Sahlgrenska University Hospital, Gothenburg, Sweden.

Mehrabi A., Department of General Surgery, Ruprecht-Karls, University of Heidelberg, Im Neuenheimer Feld 110 (Kirschnerstr. 1), D-69120 Heidelberg, Germany.

Moradpour D., Department of Medicine II, University of Freiburg, Hugstetter strasse 55, D-79106 Freiburg, Germany.

Poynard Th., Service d'Hépato-Gastroentérologie, Groupe Hospitalier Pitié-Salpêtrière, 47-83, boulevard de l'Hôpital, 75651 Paris Cedex 13.

Ratziu V., Service d'Hépato-Gastroentérologie, Groupe Hospitalier Pitié-Salpêtrière, 47-83, boulevard de l'Hôpital, 75651 Paris Cedex 13.

Schemmer P., Department of General Surgery, Ruprecht-Karls, University of Heidelberg, Im Neuenheimer Feld 110 (Kirschnerstr. 1), D-69120 Heidelberg, Germany.

Schölmerich J., Department of Internal Medicine I, University Medical Center Regensburg, D-93042 Regensburg, Germany.

Schreiber S., Ist Department of medicine, Christian-Albrechts-University, Schittenhelmstr. 12, D-24105 Kiel, Germany.

Tempia-Caliera A.A., Department of General Surgery, Ruprecht-Karls, University of Heidelberg, Im Neuenheimer Feld 110 (Kirschnerstr. 1), D-69120 Heidelberg, Germany.

New drug developments in gastroesophageal reflux disease

Jean Paul Galmiche

Department of Gastroenterology and Hepatology and CIC-INSERM, Hôtel-Dieu, Nantes, France

What is the rationale for drug development in gastroesophageal reflux disease?

During the last decade, the treatment of gastroesophageal reflux disease (GERD) was revolutionized by the rapid development of proton pump inhibitors (PPIs), which are active across the entire disease spectrum and provide more effective and rapid relief of symptoms and healing of esophagitis than any previous class of drugs used [1]. Moreover, different long-term strategies for acid suppression have been tested successfully, including continuous maintenance, intermittent and on-demand therapies [2]. However, despite these impressive advances, it is quite clear that not all the therapeutic requirements of GERD have been met [3]. First, acid suppression is unable to cure the disease, and relapses occur frequently after discontinuation of PPI therapy, mainly because underlying motor abnormalities remain unchanged after esophagitis is healed [4]. Secondly, although acid reflux is the most frequent cause of heartburn and mucosal damage, various types of refluxate exist, including solids and liquids, gas and non-acid material [5, 6]. Our understanding of the role of these non-acid components of reflux material is still limited, but may prove important in the future to explain symptoms such as extraesophageal manifestations, which are generally much more resistant to PPI therapy than heartburn [7]. With respect to the pathogenesis of GERD, several important considerations have emerged in recent years: (i) in the large majority of GERD patients, there is no mucosal break at endoscopy [8, 9], and sometimes even no excess acid reflux [10], which indicates the importance of the still poorly known influence of visceral sensitivity to different chemical or mechanical stimuli; (ii) with respect to motility disturbances, transient lower esophageal sphincter relaxations (TLESRs) represent the main underlying mechanism of reflux episodes and are a major target for drug development in endoscopy-negative GERD and in patients with mild esophagitis, although the role of other factors seems equally important in patients with hiatus hernia and/or moderate to severe esophagitis [11]; and (iii) the relation between an individual's genetic background and environmental factors is likely to be important and may account for different phenotypic responses in terms of inflammation, risk of metaplasia and ultimately adenocarcinoma of the esophagus [12, 13].

In summary, there is a rationale for drug development in GERD, and it is crucial to recognize that acid control is not the only potential target. Acid suppression is not optimal at the present time, and new PPIs are being developed to overcome the limitations of the first generation of this drug class, which could account for the failure of PPI therapy in a substantial proportion of patients *(Table I)*.

Table I. Limitations of currently used PPIs: why PPI therapy may fail in a GERD patient

---
Variable drug absorption and bioavailability between subjects
Slow onset of action
Rapid metabolism (dependence on cytochrome P450 isoenzymes)
Hypersecretor status
Nocturnal acid breakthrough
Eradication of *Helicobacter pylori*
True PPI resistance (gastric pH less than 4.0 for more than 50% of 24 h) and dosing limitations

---

Adapted from Vigneri *et al.* [14]

Ways to improve acid suppression in gastroesophageal reflux disease

All PPIs currently used in GERD are able to reduce gastric acidity dramatically during the daytime, especially after meals, but are less effective at night [15]. Nocturnal acid breakthrough (NAB, defined as a fall in gastric pH below 4.0 for at least one hour) probably has little (if any) influence on the large majority of patients whose symptoms are effectively relieved and whose esophagitis is healed by a standard once-daily morning dose of PPI (*e.g.* omeprazole 20 mg, lansoprazole 30 mg, or rabeprazole 20 mg). However, in patients with more severe disease, especially Barrett's esophagus, NAB seems to occur more frequently and is more likely to be accompanied by esophageal acidification [16]. Therefore, a better control of nocturnal acid secretion would appear to be a rational approach for these patients (*for a review, see* [17]). In acute experiments, a twice-daily dose of omeprazole and ranitidine proved effective [18], although a recent study has shown that tolerance to H_2-blockers develops rapidly [19], preventing any significant benefit from this combined therapy after one week of continuous administration. Despite a lack of any significant benefit for an average group of GERD patients, it is noteworthy that some individuals continue to respond to this form of acid suppression well beyond one week. Thus, it is important to individualize therapy in severe GERD and to check for continued acid suppression by repeated 24-h gastric pH-monitoring in patients undergoing treatment for at least several weeks or months. The potential benefit of aggressive acid suppression in Barrett's esophagus may have different biological and molecular aspects, *e.g.* reduction of acid-induced cell proliferation, reduction of duodeno-gastroesophageal (bile) reflux, decreased cyclooxygenase-2 (COX-2) expression and PGE2 release, and suppression of acid-induced activation of mitogen-activated protein kinase pathways [20].

Are new PPIs more effective in GERD patients?

The good results for esomeprazole, the S-enantiomer of omeprazole, indicate that better acid suppression provides clinical benefits in terms of symptom relief and healing of esophagitis, especially in severe cases (*for a review, see* [14]). However, NAB still occurs with the standard 40 mg dose, and no results seem to be available for higher dosages or dosing frequencies (*e.g.* 40 mg b.i.d.). Other PPIs are currently under development, and preliminary results suggest that control of nocturnal acidity is improved with tenatoprazole (unpublished data). The clinical relevance of more prolonged acid suppression, notably for regression of metaplasia and dysplasia and thus reduction of cancer risk, remains to be determined. Although attempts in some pilot studies to abolish distal acid exposure resulted in a decrease of 1 to 3 cm in the length of Barrett's mucosa [21], there is evidence that the risk of esophageal adenocarcinoma remains increased, even after antireflux surgery [22].

Which drugs can be used to correct motility disturbances?

GERD is frequently associated with motor disturbances that are not limited to the lower esophageal sphincter (LES), but include defective esophageal peristalsis, resulting in impaired clearance, enhanced postprandial gastric relaxation (which may trigger TLESRs) and delayed gastric emptying. A prokinetic drug acts either directly on smooth muscle or on the myenteric plexus [23]. Unfortunately, most of the prokinetics previously used in GERD have not proved to be very effective (*e.g.* metoclopramide and domperidone) or have been associated with unacceptable side effects (*e.g.* metoclopramide and cisapride). One reason for the disappointing results of cisapride may be that prokinetic effects wane with chronic use. Indeed, a recent work by Finizia *et al.* [24] failed to detect any effect of cisapride 20 mg b.i.d. on esophageal motility parameters and TLESRs (induced by gastric distension) after 4 weeks of therapy in GERD patients. These data are in agreement with the results of another study showing that cisapride (10 mg qds) had no effect on 24-h esophageal motility, LES pressure and the incidence of TLESRs after one week of treatment in GERD patients [25].

New pharmacological approaches recently explored for the treatment of GERD correspond not only to different classes of drugs, including prokinetic substances such as motilin agonists (*i.e.* motilides) and 5-hydroxytryptamine (5-HT) receptor agonists, but also (and more importantly) to a group of agents sometimes referred to as "eukinetics" [3] or "anti-relaxation therapy" [26], because they are mainly intended to modulate TLESRs [27]. TLESRs are indeed the most important underlying motor mechanism responsible for acid and non-acid reflux episodes, especially in endoscopy-negative GERD and mild esophagitis.

Intravenous erythromycin was initially reported to increase LES pressure and esophageal motility as well as to accelerate gastric emptying and enhance proximal gastric tone in healthy volunteers and GERD patients [28-31]. However, other studies found that oral erythromycin was ineffective in GERD patients [32]. Now that the motilin receptor has been cloned, the development of motilides (*i.e.* motilin agonists without antibiotic properties) has received considerable attention. However, despite their accelerating effects on gastric emptying and their ability to increase LES pressure in animals [33], the therapeutic potential of motilides in GERD seems very limited or even inconsequential. A recent study [25] conducted in patients with heartburn showed that motilin agonist ABT 229 (5 mg and 10 mg b.i.d. given orally for 7 days) had no effect on acid exposure or esophageal motility (LES pressure and incidence of TLESRs). However, for undetermined reasons, the severity of daytime heartburn was slightly, but significantly, reduced (to the same magnitude as with cisapride 10 mg).

Tegaserod is a selective 5-HT4 partial agonist derived from amino guanidine indoles. Although it has been developed primarily in irritable bowel syndrome, a recent pharmacological crossover study explored its potential usefulness in GERD [34]. Four doses of tegaserod (1, 4, 12 and 24 mg twice daily) and placebo were tested in GERD patients to assess the dose-response effect on esophageal acid exposure and LES motility. The results indicated a slight, but statistically significant, reduction of esophageal acid exposure during the postprandial period, with no significant effect on LES pressure or TLESRs (only a trend to reduction of the latter). Similarly, a decreased, but not statistically significant, number of reflux episodes was reported. Clearly, these results, which were obtained with the lower doses (1 and 4 mg) of tegaserod tested, are not very impressive and were not reproduced with the higher doses (12 and 24 mg). Despite the excellent tolerance obtained for doses of < 12 mg b.i.d., these preliminary results clearly require confirmation before a clinical trial is conducted. The possibility of desensitization of 5-HT-4 receptors with higher doses or of recruitment of other 5-HT receptors with opposite effects also limits the potential usefulness of this drug in a disease such as GERD in which titration and individualization of therapy are frequently required. The effects of tegaserod on TLESRs need to be confirmed, as other 5-HT receptors may be involved, especially 5-HT-3 [35].

As indicated above, the last but probably most promising pharmacological approach consists in developing drugs specifically targeted to TLESRs [36]. Theoretically, several drugs are pharmacologically active on TLESRs *(Table II)*, but the clinical use of many of them in GERD is precluded by their broader effects on GI motility and/or other extradigestive pharmacological actions *(for a review, see* [27, 37, 38]). In principle, drugs acting on the afferent loop of this vago-vagal reflex, or at the central level on the TLESR generator, are more appropriate than those acting on efferent pathways. Indeed, intervention on efferent pathways may result in a situation comparable to achalasia, with impairment of normal swallow-induced LES relaxations.

Table II. List of drugs shown to reduce the incidence of transient LES relaxations in animals, or humans, or both

Anticholinergics (atropine)
Morphine
Cholecystokinin (CCK)1 antagonists (devazepide and loxiglumide)
Serotonin (5-HT3) antagonists (ondansetron and granisetron)
Nitric oxide synthase inhibitors (L-NAME and L-NMMA)
Somatostatin
NMDA (riluzole)
$GABA_B$ agonists (baclofen)
Lidocaine

Adapted from Hirsch *et al.* [37] and Holloway [27]

Although atropine and morphine are extremely effective in reducing the incidence of TLESRs (most likely through a central effect) [39], their clinical potential in GERD is probably limited because of the risk of poor tolerance and side effects, unless more specific agonists/antagonists are developed. The same holds true for inhibitors of nitric oxide synthesis.

As cholecystokinin (CCK) plays an important role in the triggering of TLESRs [40], the therapeutic potential of selective CCK-1 antagonists was tested in both healthy volunteers and GERD patients [41-44]. Loxiglumide, the most promising compound, reduces the fall in LES pressure following a meal and dramatically inhibits the incidence of postprandial TLESRs *(Figure 1)*, an effect that may also be related to marked inhibition of proximal gastric relaxation [42]. Unfortunately, despite this interesting pharmacological profile, loxiglumide appears to have only modest effects on postprandial acid exposure [45].

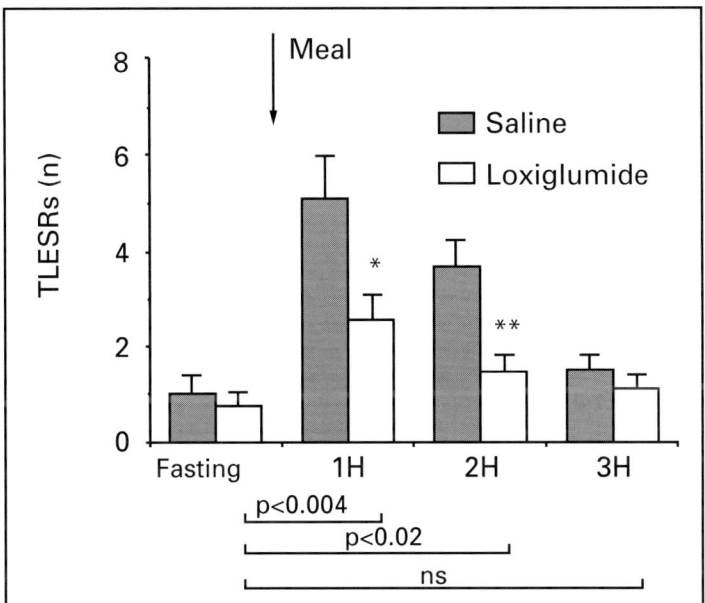

Figure 1. Inhibition of meal-induced TLESRs by the CCK1 receptor antagonist loxiglumide (reproduced with permission of *Am J Physiol* [42]).

Gamma-aminobutyric acid (GABA) is a major inhibitory transmitter within the central nervous system. $GABA_B$ receptors are present pre-synaptically on vagal afferents in the dorsal medulla, and their activation can inhibit neurotransmitter release in vagal nuclei [46]. Recently, baclofen, a $GABA_B$ agonist, was shown to reduce the number of TLESRs dramatically in ferrets, dogs and humans [47-49]. Baclofen acts primarily at the central level, but a decrease in mechano-receptor sensitivity and an increase in gastric tone may also contribute to the effects of this substance on TLESRs. In healthy human volunteers, a single oral dose of 40 mg can reduce the rate of TLESRs by approximately 50% and increase LES pressure without affecting the duration of TLESRs or residual pressure during TLESRs [47]. Zhang *et al.* [49] confirmed these effects on esophageal motility in patients with reflux esophagitis *(Figure 2)*, but failed to detect any significant decrease of postprandial esophageal acid exposure. However, their study was not designed and powered to detect a clinical benefit. Recently, Van Herwaarden *et al* [50] investigated the effect of baclofen in 37 patients with GERD. A randomized double-blind placebo controlled two-way crossover study was used and the effect of baclofen (single-dose) on symptoms was also determined during the post-prandial periods of two study days. Although these authors confirmed the effect of baclofen in reducing TLESRs and were able to detect a significant decrease of esophageal acid exposure, they could not demonstrate a benefit in terms of symptom relief. Further studies are required to explore the potential of $GABA_B$ agonists in GERD. In fact, baclofen has some advantages over other agents, namely availability in an oral formulation, current clinical applications in other indications (particularly spasticity for which it is employed at a higher dose), and no deleterious effects on esophageal acid clearance (contrary to the action of atropine or morphine). Clearly baclofen is a prototype drug, and further pharmacological research is needed to improve this type of antireflux therapy and design novel targeted compounds. In this respect, it is noteworthy that all responses to baclofen are not equally affected by $GABA_B$ antagonists, which suggests that several isoforms of receptors may be present. After the recent cloning of GABA receptors, new compounds with more specific actions may become available in the near future. It is also noteworthy that only the R enantiomer of baclofen was able

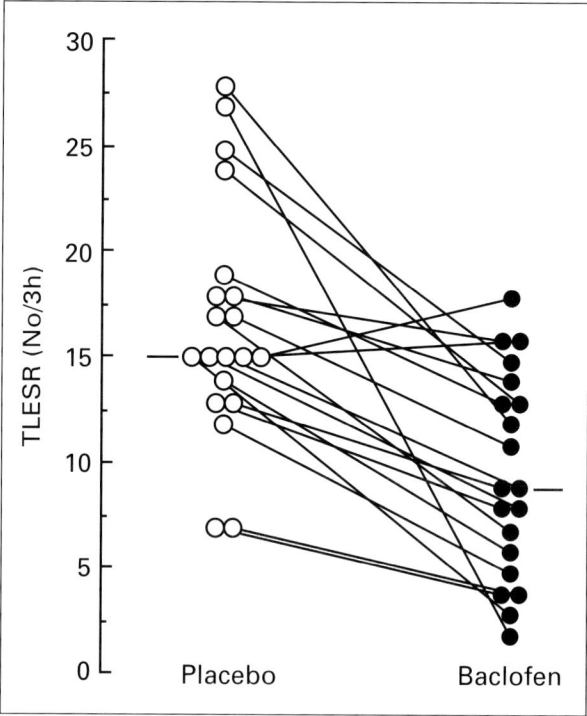

Figure 2. Inhibition of TLESRs by the $GABA_B$ agonist baclofen (40 mg orally) in GERD patients (reproduced with permission of *Gut* [49]).

to reduce the rate of TLESRs in dogs, while the S isomer was completely ineffective [48]. The pharmacological manipulation of other receptors, including somatostatin and glutamate receptors (*e.g.* NMDA receptors), remains to be explored [37].

Although it is unlikely that anti-relaxation therapy will replace PPIs in moderate or severe GERD, eukinetics may be applicable to patients with mild disease and/or to children, as pediatricians are usually reluctant to consider very prolonged (lifetime?) acid suppression in this group of patients. Anti-relaxation therapy may be useful as well, not only as an alternative to acid suppression, but also as an add-on therapy in patients with severe disease and in those with incomplete response to PPIs or non-acid (biliary) reflux. As recently indicated by Holloway [27], "we are only on the threshold of transition from concept to a practical stage".

Possible means of reducing inflammation and controlling proliferation/differentiation in reflux esophagitis and Barrett's esophagus

Although the majority of GERD patients do not have mucosal breaks or exhibit only minimal inflammation at endoscopy, some experience more severe esophagitis, or complications, or both. These patients may be difficult to manage even with very potent acid suppression, because other factors than acid contribute to the pathogenesis of the disease. For example, bile acids seem to play a significant role in Barrett's esophagus, thus increasing the risk of dysplasia and malignant transformation. Therefore, other pharmacological approaches than pure reduction of acid exposure may prove beneficial, *e.g.* those related to the potential of anti-inflammatory compounds and substances to regulate proliferation and differentiation within the esophageal mucosa [51]. These molecular and biochemical strategies have only recently been explored in GERD, but some data are promising for the development of chemoprophylaxis of adenocarcinoma.

Antioxidants such as DA 9601 have been tested in animal models. For example, Oh *et al.* [52] recently reported that this compound was able to attenuate inflammation in a rat model of esophagitis induced by mixed (acidic and biliary) reflux. It was more effective than ranitidine, but unfortunately the authors did not compare its efficacy with that of a PPI. The mechanism of action, which was at least partly deciphered, involves the NFkB transcription factor pathway.

COX-2 (prostaglandin synthase 2) may be an important target for chemoprophylaxis, as it plays an important role in cell growth and differentiation [52]. COX-2 expression has been induced by several stimuli in various animal inflammation models and in inflammatory human diseases. It is implicated in colorectal, gastric and esophageal carcinogenesis. In Barrett's esophagus there is a progressive increase in COX-2 levels from metaplasia to dysplasia and adenocarcinoma. In *ex vivo* studies using Barrett's explants, it was demonstrated that pulses of acid or bile acids upregulate COX2 expression. Kaur *et al.* [53] recently reported a significant reduction of COX2 expression in 12 patients with Barrett's esophagus after 10 days of oral therapy with the selective COX2 inhibitor rofecoxib at a daily dose of 25 mg. PGE2 and PCNA (a proliferation marker) were also significantly reduced. Although the rationale for this approach seems reasonable, additional data and more prolonged studies are needed to determine whether rofecoxib is useful or not in preventing dysplasia and cancer in Barrett's esophagus *(Figure 3)*.

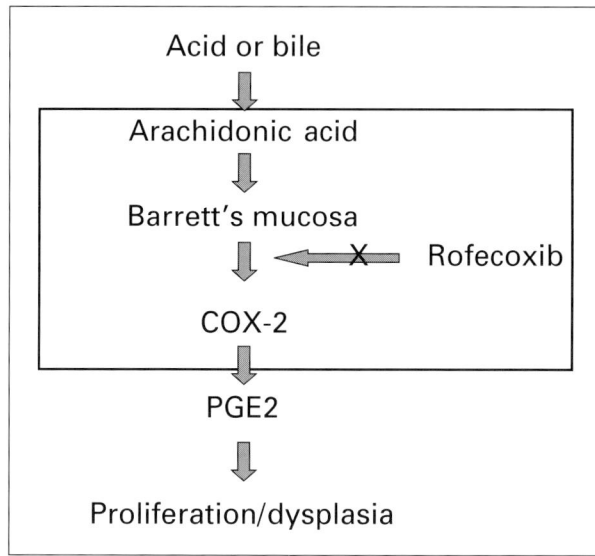

Figure 3. Hypothetical model outlining the proliferation mechanism in Barrett's esophagus exposed to acid or bile in the refluxate, with potential implications for the risk of dysplasia. COX-2 inhibition therapy with rofecoxib reduces COX-2 expression, PGE2 production and proliferation (reproduced with permission of *Gastroenterology* [53]).

Summary and conclusions

1. Acid suppression with current PPIs is not optimal in GERD, as NAB frequently occurs and may be particularly relevant in Barrett's esophagus or severe GERD. The combination of a PPI with an H2-receptor antagonist provides effective control of nocturnal acid secretion, but the rapid development of tolerance to H2-receptor antagonist probably makes this therapy less useful than initially expected. Research on new PPIs (*i.e.* irreversible or reversible PPIs) is still in progress.

2. TLESRs are the main underlying mechanism of both acid and non-acid reflux episodes in endoscopy-negative GERD and mild esophagitis and are therefore a major therapeutic target for new drug developments. Various drugs can be effective in reducing the incidence of TLESRs, but their therapeutic use in GERD is precluded by non-specific actions and potential (unacceptable) side effects. The most promising agents in this area are $GABA_B$ agonists, with oral baclofen as a prototype drug. Determination of the benefit of oral therapy with baclofen or its derivative requires further studies specifically designed for measurement of 24-h acid exposure and clinically relevant endpoints, not only after acute administration but also in conditions of chronic use.

3. As chronic GERD and Barrett's esophagus expose patients to increased risk of dysplasia and adenocarcinoma of the esophagus, there is a rationale for development of chemoprophylaxis. Preliminary data with COX-2 inhibitors are encouraging, but need confirmation.

4. Drug therapy should be compared with other antireflux strategies including surgery and endoscopic approaches.

References

1. Chiba N, De Gara CJ, Wilkinson JM. Speed of healing and symptom relief in grade II to IV gastroesophageal reflux disease: a meta-analysis. *Gastroenterology* 1997; 112: 1798-810.
2. Talley NJ, Venables TL, Green JR, Armstrong D, O'Kane KP, Giaffer M, *et al*. Esomeprazole 40 mg and 20 mg is efficacious in the long-term management of patients with endoscopy-negative gastro-oesophageal reflux disease: a placebo-controlled trial of on-demand therapy for 6 months. *Eur J Gastroenterol Hepatol* 2002; 14: 857-63.
3. Dent J. Gastro-oesophageal reflux disease. *Digestion* 1998; 59: 433-45.
4. Singh P, Adamopoulos A, Taylor RH, Colin-Jones DG. Oesophageal motor function before and after healing of oesophagitis. *Gut* 1992; 33: 1590-6.
5. Sifrim D, Holloway R, Silny J. Acid, nonacid, and gas reflux in patients with gastroesophageal reflux disease during ambulatory 24-hour pH-impedance recordings. *Gastroenterology* 2001; 120: 1588-98.
6. Vela MF, Camacho-Lobato L. Srinivasan R. Simultaneous intraesophageal impedance and pH measurement of acid and nonacid gastroesophageal reflux: effect of omeprazole. *Gastroenterology* 2001; 120: 1599-606.
7. Kahrilas PJ. Management of GERD: medical *versus* surgical. *Semin Gastrointest Dis* 2001; 12: 3-15.
8. Galmiche JP, Barthélémy P, Hamelin B. Treating the symptoms of gastro-oesophageal reflux disease: a double-blind comparison of omeprazole and cisapride. *Aliment Pharmacol Ther* 1997; 11: 765-73.
9. Galmiche JP, Bruley des Varannes S. Endoscopy-negative reflux disease. *Curr Gastroenterol Rep* 2001; 3: 206-14.
10. Shi G, Bruley des Varannes S, Scarpignato C, Le Rhun M, Galmiche JP. Reflux-related symptoms in patients with normal oesophageal exposure to acid. *Gut* 1995; 37: 457-64.
11. Van Herwaarden MA, Samsom M, Smout AJPM. Excess gastroesophageal reflux in patients with hiatus hernia is caused by mechanisms other than transient LES relaxations. *Gastroenterology* 2000; 119: 1439-46.
12. Fitzgerald RC, Onwuegbusi BA, Bajaj-Elliott M, Saeed IT, Burnham WR, Farthing MJG. Diversity in the oesophageal phenotypic response to gastro-oesophageal reflux: immunological determinants. *Gut* 2002; 50: 451-9.
13. Romero Y, Locke GR. Is there a GERD gene? *Am J Gastroenterol* 1999; 94: 1127-8.
14. Vigneri S, Tonini M, Scarpignato C, Savarino V. Improving opportunities for effective management of gastro-oesophageal reflux disease. *Digest Liver Dis* 2001; 33: 719-29.
15. Peghini PL, Katz PO, Bracy NA, Castell DO. Nocturnal recovery of gastric acid secretion with twice-daily dosing of proton pump inhibitors. *Am J Gastroenterol* 1998; 93: 763-7.
16. Katz PO, Anderson C, Khoury R, Castell DO. Gastro-oesophageal reflux associated with nocturnal gastric acid breakthrough on proton pump inhibitors. *Aliment Pharmacol Ther* 1998; 12: 1231-4.
17. Fitzgerald RC, Lascar R, Triadafilopoulos G. Review article: Barrett's oesophagus, dysplasia and pharmacologic acid suppression. *Aliment Pharmacol Ther* 2001; 15: 269-76.
18. Peghini PL, Katz PO, Castell DO. Ranitidine controls nocturnal gastric acid breakthrough on omeprazole: a controlled study in normal subjects. *Gastroenterology* 1998; 115: 1335-9.

19. Fackler WK, Ours TM, Vaezi MF, Richter JE. Long-term effect of H2RA therapy on nocturnal gastric acid breakthrough. *Gastroenterology* 2002; 122: 625-32.
20. Souza RF, Shewmake K, Terada LS, Spechler SJ. Acid exposure activates the mitogen-activated protein kinase pathways in Barrett's esophagus. *Gastroenterology* 2002; 122: 299-307.
21. Srinivasan R, Katz PO, Ramakrishnan A, Katzka DA, Vela MF, Castell DO. Maximal acid reflux control for Barrett's oesophagus: feasible and effective. *Aliment Pharmacol Ther* 2001; 15: 519-24.
22. Ye W, Chow WH, Lagergren J, Yin L, Nyren O. Risk of adenocarcinomas of the esophagus and gastric cardia in patients with gastroesophageal reflux diseases and after antireflux surgery. *Gastroenterology* 2001; 121: 1286-93.
23. De Caestecker J. Prokinetics and reflux: a promise unfulfilled. *Eur J Gastroenterol Hepatol* 2002; 14: 5-7.
24. Finizia C, Lundell L, Cange L, Ruth M. The effect of cisapride on oesophageal motility and lower sphincter function in patients with gastro-oesophageal reflux disease. *Eur J Gastroenterol Hepatol* 2002; 14: 9-14.
25. Van Herwaarden MA, Samsom M, Van Nispen CHM, Verlinden M, Smout AJP. The effect of motilin agonist ABT-229 on gastro-oesophageal reflux, oesophageal motility and lower oesophageal sphincter characteristics in GERD patients. *Aliment Pharmacol Ther* 2000; 14: 453-62.
26. Tack J, Sifrim D. Anti-relaxation therapy in GORD. *Gut* 2002; 50: 6-7.
27. Holloway RH. Systemic pharmacomodulation of transient lower esophageal sphincter relaxations. *Am J Med* 2001; 111: 178S-85S.
28. Chaussade S, Michopoulos S, Sogni P, Guerre J, Couturier D. Motilin agonist erythromycin increases human lower esophageal sphincter pressure by stimulation of cholinergic nerves. *Dig Dis Sci* 1994; 39: 381-4.
29. Chrysos E, Tzovaras G, Epanomeritakis E, Tsiaoussis J, Vrachasotakis N, Vassilakid JS, Xynos E. Erythromycin enhances oesophageal motility in patients with gastro-oesophageal reflux. *ANZ J Surg* 2001; 71: 98-102.
30. Tzovaras G, Xynos E, Chrysos E, Mantides A, Vassilakis JS. The effect of intravenous erythromycin on esophageal motility in healthy subjects. *Am J Surg* 1996; 171: 316-9.
31. Bruley des Varannes S, Parys V, Ropert A, Chayvialle JA, Rozé C, Galmiche JP. Erythromycin enhances fasting and postprandial proximal gastric tone in humans. *Gastroenterology* 1995; 109: 32-9.
32. Champion G, Richter JE, Singh S, Schan C, Nellans H. Effects of oral erythromycin on esophageal pH and pressure profiles in patients with gastroesophageal reflux disease. *Dig Dis Sci* 1994; 39: 129-37.
33. Greenwood B, Dieckman D, Kirst HA, Gidda JS. Effects of LY267108, an erythromycin analogue derivative, on lower esophageal sphincter function in the cat. *Gastroenterology* 1994; 106: 624-8.
34. Kahrilas PJ, Quigley EMM, Castell DO, Spechler S. The effects of tegaserod (HTF 919) on oesophageal acid exposure in gastro-oesophageal reflux disease. *Aliment Pharmacol Ther* 2000; 14: 1503-9.
35. Rouzade ML, Fioramonti J, Buéno L. Rôle des récepteurs 5-HT3 dans le contrôle par la cholécystokinine des relaxations transitoires du sphincter inférieur de l'œsophage chez le chien. *Gastroenterol Clin Biol* 1996; 20: 575-80.
36. Janssens J, Sifrim D. Spontaneous transient lower esophageal sphincter relaxations: a target for treatment of gastroesophageal reflux disease. *Gastroenterology* 1995; 109: 1703-5.
37. Hirsch DP, Tytgat GNJ, Boeckxstaens GEE. Review article: transient lower oesophageal sphincter relaxations – a pharmacological target for gastro-oesophageal reflux disease? *Aliment Pharmacol Ther* 2002; 16: 17-26.
38. Galmiche JP, Zerbib F. Mechanisms of gastro-oesophageal reflux disease (GORD) and potential targets for anti-reflux therapy. In: Farthing MJG, Bianchi Porro G, eds. *New horizons in gastrointestinal and liver disease: mechanisms and management*. Paris: John Libbey Eurotext, 1999: 3-15.

39. Penagini R, Bianchi PA. Effect of morphine on gastroesophageal reflux and transient lower esophageal sphincter relaxation. *Gastroenterology* 1997; 113: 409-14.
40. Boulant J, Fioramonti J, Dapoigny M, Bommelaer G, Bueno L. Cholecystokinin and nitric oxide in transient lower esophageal sphincter relaxation to gastric distension in dogs. *Gastroenterology* 1994; 107: 1059-66.
41. Boulant J, Mathieu S, D'Amato M, Abergel A, Dapoigny M, Bommelaer G. Cholecystokinin in transient lower oesophageal sphincter relaxation due to gastric distension in humans. *Gut* 1997; 40: 575-81.
42. Zerbib F, Bruley des Varannes S, Scarpignato C, Leray V, D'Amato M, Rozé C, Galmiche JP. Endogenous cholecystokinin in postprandial lower esophageal sphincter function and fundic tone in humans. *Am J Physiol* 1998; 38: G1266-G1273.
43. Clavé P, Gonzalez A, Moreno A, Lopez R, Farré A, Cusso X, D'Amato M, Azpiroz F, Lluis F. Endogenous cholecystokinin enhances postprandial gastroesophageal reflux in humans through extrasphincteric receptors. *Gastroenterology* 1998; 115: 597-604.
44. Boeckxstaens GE, Hirsch DP, Fakhry N, Holloway RH, D'Amato M, Tytgat GNJ. Involvement of cholecystokinin receptors in transient lower esophageal sphincter relaxations triggered by gastric distension. *Am J Gastroenterol* 1998; 93: 1823-8.
45. Trudgill NJ, Hussain FN, Moustafa M, Ajjan MR, D'Amato M, Riley SA. The effect of cholecystokinin antagonism on postprandial lower oesophageal sphincter function in asymptomatic volunteers and patients with reflux disease. *Aliment Pharmacol Ther* 2001; 15: 1357-64.
46. Blackshaw LA. Receptors and transmission in the brain-gut axis: potential for novel therapies. *Am J Physiol Gastrointest Liver Physiol* 2001; 281: G311-G315.
47. Lidums I, Lehmann A, Checklin H, Dent J, Holloway RH. Control of transient lower esophageal sphincter relaxations and reflux by the $GABA_B$ agonist baclofen in normal subjects. *Gastroenterology* 2000; 118: 7-13.
48. Lehmann A, Antonsson M, Bremner-Danielsen M, Flärdh M, Hansson-Bränden L, Kärrberg L. Activation of the $GABA_B$ receptor inhibits transient lower esophageal sphincter relaxations in dogs. *Gastroenterology* 1999; 117: 1147-54.
49. Zhang Q, Lehmann A, Rigda R, Dent J, Holloway RH. Control of transient lower oesophageal sphincter relaxations and reflux by the $GABA_B$ agonist baclofen in patients with gastro-oesophageal reflux disease. *Gut* 2002; 50: 19-24.
50. Van Herwaarden MA, Samsom M, Rydholm H, Smout AJPM. The effect of baclofen on gastro-oesophageal reflux, lower oesophageal sphincter function and reflux symptoms in patients with reflux disease. *Aliment Pharmacol Ther* 2002; 16: 1655-62.
51. Fitzgerald RC. Beyond acid suppressants in gastro-oesophageal reflux disease. *Gut* 2001; 49: 320-1.
52. Oh TY, Lee JS, Ahn BO, Cho H, Kim WB, Surh YJ, et al. Oxidative stress is more important than acid in the pathogenesis of reflux. *Gut* 2001; 49: 364-71.
53. Kaur BS, Khamnehei N, Iravani M, Namburu SS, Lin O, Triadafilopoulos G. Rofecoxib inhibits cyclooxygenase 2 expression and activity and reduces cell proliferation in Barrett's esophagus. *Gastroenterology* 2002; 123: 60-7.

Basic Mechanisms of Digestive Diseases: the Rationale for Clinical Management and Prevention.
M.J.G. Farthing, P. Malfertheiner, eds. John Libbey Eurotext, Paris © 2002, pp. 13-22.

Advances in treatment strategies for gastroesophageal reflux disease

Lars Lundell

Department of Surgery, Sahlgrenska University Hospital, Gothenburg, Sweden

Gastroesophageal reflux disease (GERD) can broadly be defined as troublesome symptoms which occur as a consequence of reflux of gastric juice into the oesophagus with or without oesophageal mucosa damage. This is a frequent and wide spread disorder particularly in the Western societies. It can be calculated that about 25 millions US citizens experience reflux daily. Since negative health consequences of reflux disease are rare, the major impact of the disease follows the function of the symptom burden and the impact of the symptoms on health related sense of wellbeing. Heartburn is the most prevalent symptom of GERD and it follows that the health related sense of wellbeing is impaired in proportion to the frequency and severity of heartburn. Heartburn frequency does become an important facet of the operational definition upon which the diagnostic evaluation must attempt to establish [1-4]. The introduction of the proton pump inhibitor (PPI) represents an enormous therapeutic advantage for reflux disease. Even when a treatment option has been defined by a series of clinical trials, the use of PPIs in clinical practice usually requires further refinement. This is particularly so when there are several options for management of the same disease as in the case of GERD. Symptoms frequency and intensity are the most important measures of severity of GERD and will support the treatment aim of symptom relief. Patients enrolled in clinical trials, who had troublesome reflux symptoms, but no endoscopic evidence of oesophagitis, showed a similar distribution of severity of heartburn compared with patients with severe oesophagitis. Consequently, oesophagitis and symptoms severity should be taken as independent and equally important measures of severity of the disease and therefore assessed separately [4].

Initial management

Abolition of abnormal oesophageal acid exposure is a powerful predictor of successful treatment of reflux disease [5, 6]. This information may assist in the management of individual patients in whom the cause of symptoms is unclear and normalisation of acid exposure during therapy indicates successful treatment *(Figure 1)*. It should be noted that control of oesophageal acid exposure cannot always be achieved with standard doses on PPIs, as a minority of patients will require higher doses. A therapeutic test with PPIs is an useful option for assistance with diagnosis provided that a careful symptom analysis suggests reflux disease [7, 8]. Furthermore, a therapeutic test can also be helpful for recognition of reflux-induced hoarseness and asthma and in patients with non-cardiac chest pain [9]. The effectiveness of the therapeutic test depends on the introduction of acid inhibition which is strong enough to abolish or almost completely prevent acid reflux and the continuation of treatment for a time period which is long enough to ascertain whether the symptoms have been resolved or at least substantially improved [10, 11]. The PPI-based therapeutic test has been shown to be slightly more sensitive than pH monitoring despite the fact that the chosen doses were probably not sufficiently high to achieve optimal results in terms of acid inhibition. A recent trial evaluated the diagnostic value of the confirmatory test by use of esomeprazole in patients with suspected GERD. The sensitivity of confirming GERD for the two esomeprazole regimens increased during the first treatment days and stabilised between 79% and 86% after the five-day treatment. Thus treatment test with esomeprazole 40 mg has a high sensitivity in confirming GERD [12].

Long-term treatment by medical therapies

Reflux disease is usually a significant recurrent problem if the pretreatment symptoms are troublesome enough to cause disability and impaired quality of life. In patients with relatively severe oesophagitis, withdrawal of short-term therapy has been associated with symptomatic and endoscopic relapse in most patients. The response to short-term PPI treatment has proved to be a reliable predictor of the efficacy of a long-term treatment [13]. PPIs have been shown to be effective and safe when used as maintenance therapy. Comparative trials have shown that both 20 and 10 mg of omeprazole are significantly more effective than placebo and H_2-receptors antagonists. Accordingly trials long-term therapy with for instance lanzoprazole have shown that both 30 and 15 mg daily are superior to placebo and ranitidine. In order to minimise drug exposure and cost, maintenance treatment may therefore be started with or stepped down to a lower dose of PPI given once daily *(Figure 2)*. However, the physician should be prepared to return to full dosage if relapse or symptoms indicate this dose to be suboptimal. This strategy is based on the evidence that relief from heartburn is highly predictable for maintained healing of oesophagitis. Even in patients with more severe grades of oesophagitis, PPIs in standard daily doses are adequate in all but a minority of cases and this effect can be maintained for years [14-16]. In recent trials with the new generation of isomer PPI (esomeprazole) in doses in 40 and 20 mg once daily it was interesting to observe that a more profound and sustained level of acid inhibition had an immediate impact on therapy in form of that the initial grade of oesophagitis seemed not to be prognostically important. For 20 and 40 mg daily of esomeprazole, the relapse risk was estimated to centre around 10% during a 6-12 month follow-up period. There was also a difference in how patients responded. While both doses maintained healing in the vast majority of patients, a greater proportion of patients maintained control of heartburn with the 40 mg dose. These results coincide

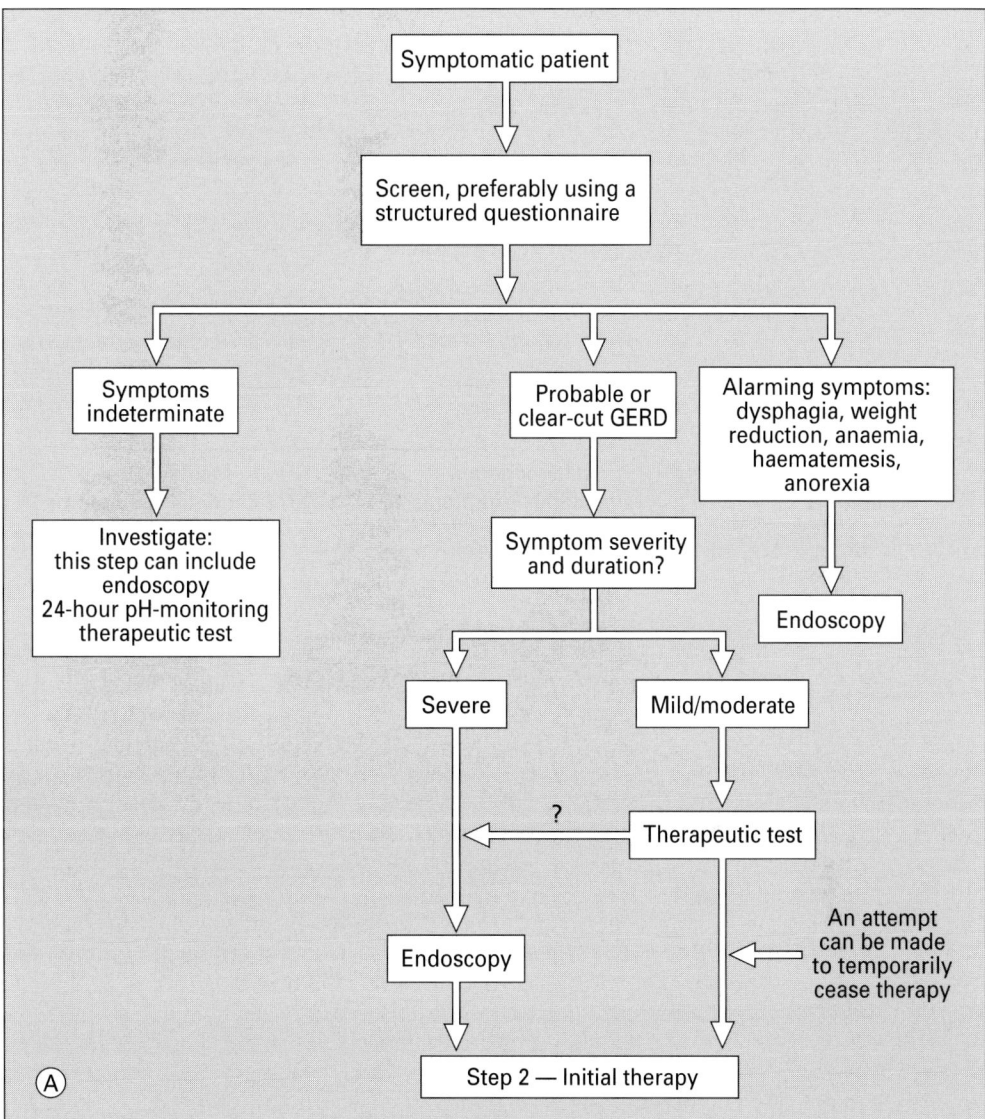

Figure 1. Management algorithm for patients with symptoms suggestive of GERD. H_2RA, H_2-receptor antagonist; PPI, proton pump inhibitor. A: Step 1; B: Step 2; C: Step 2b.

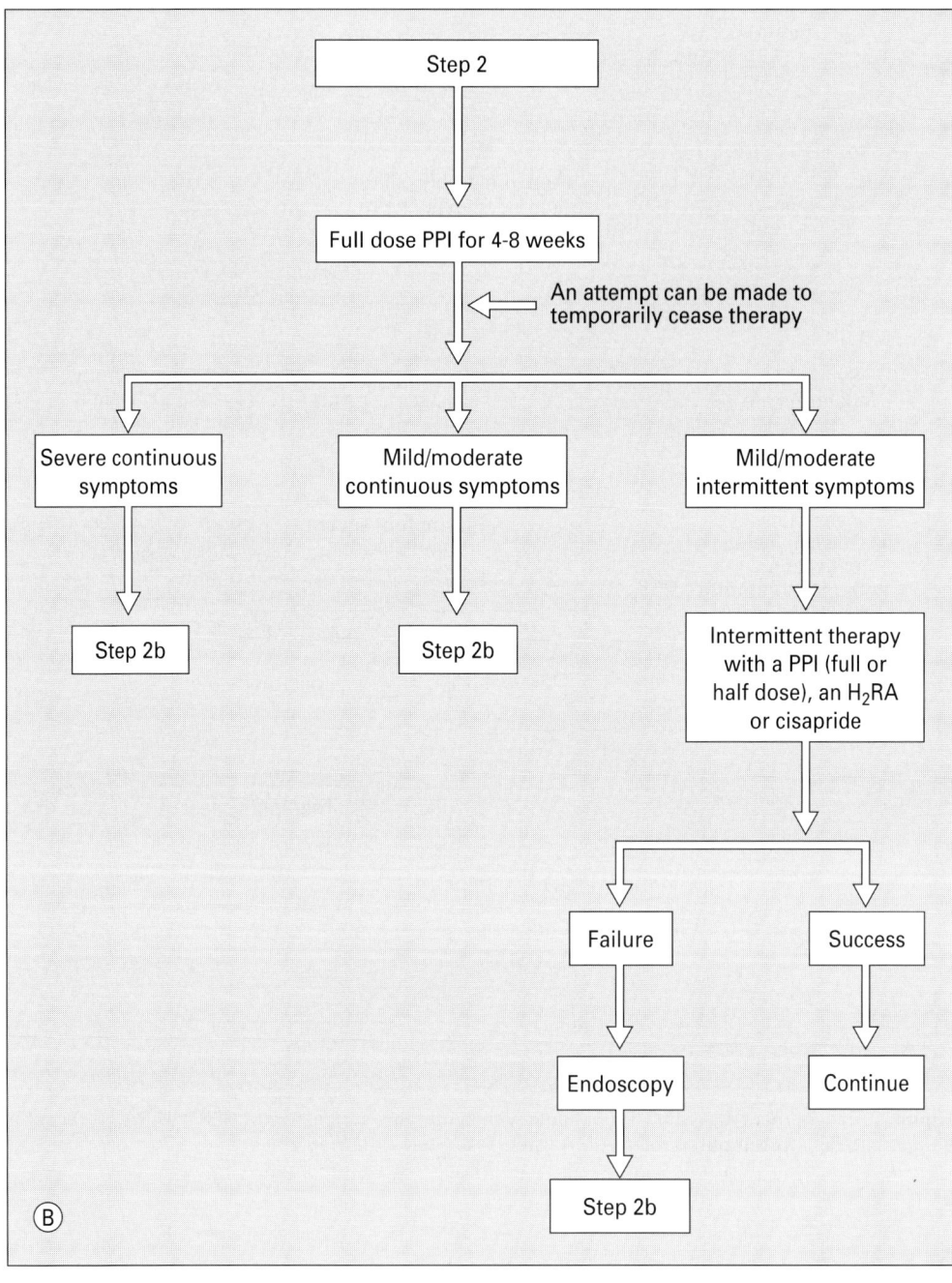

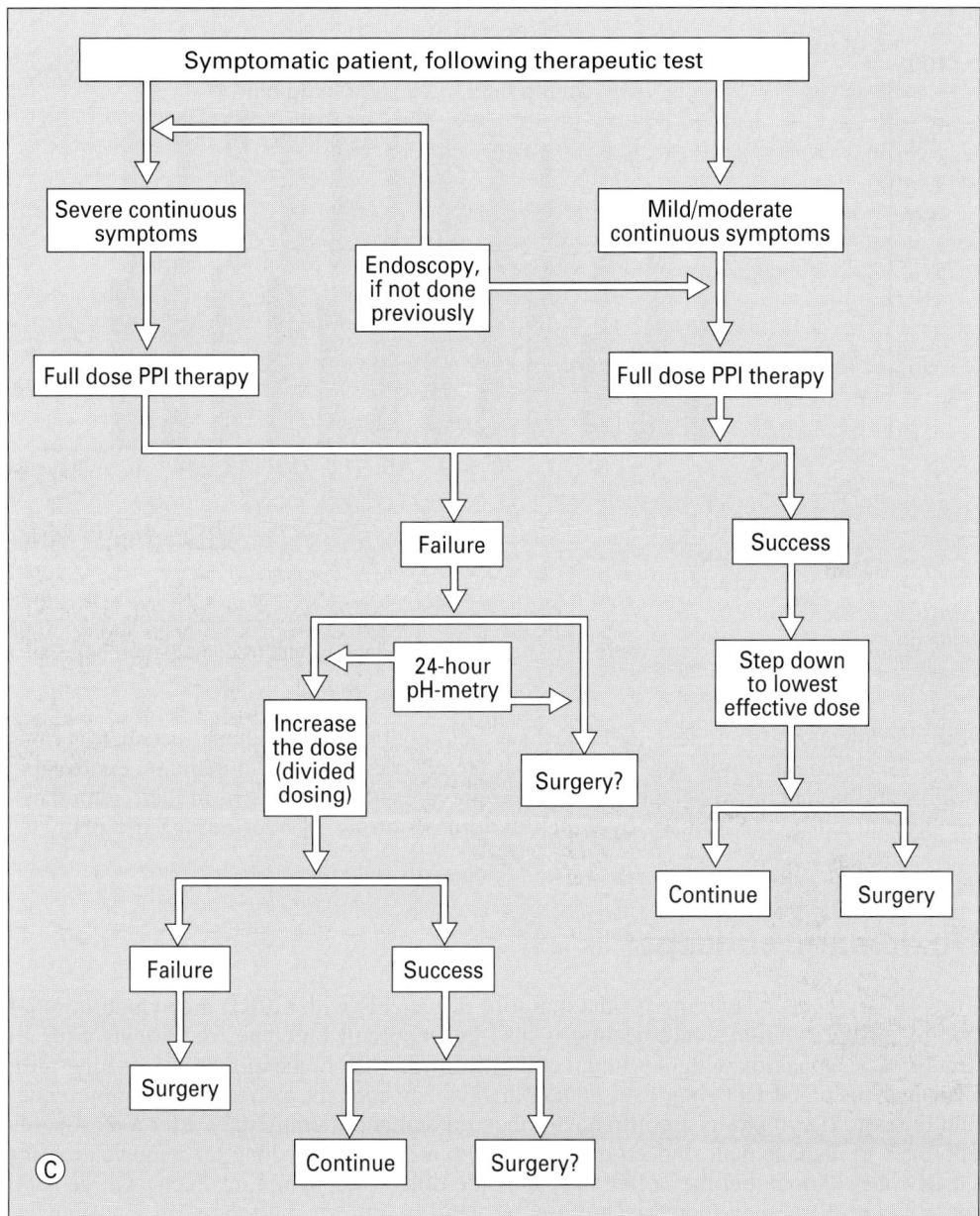

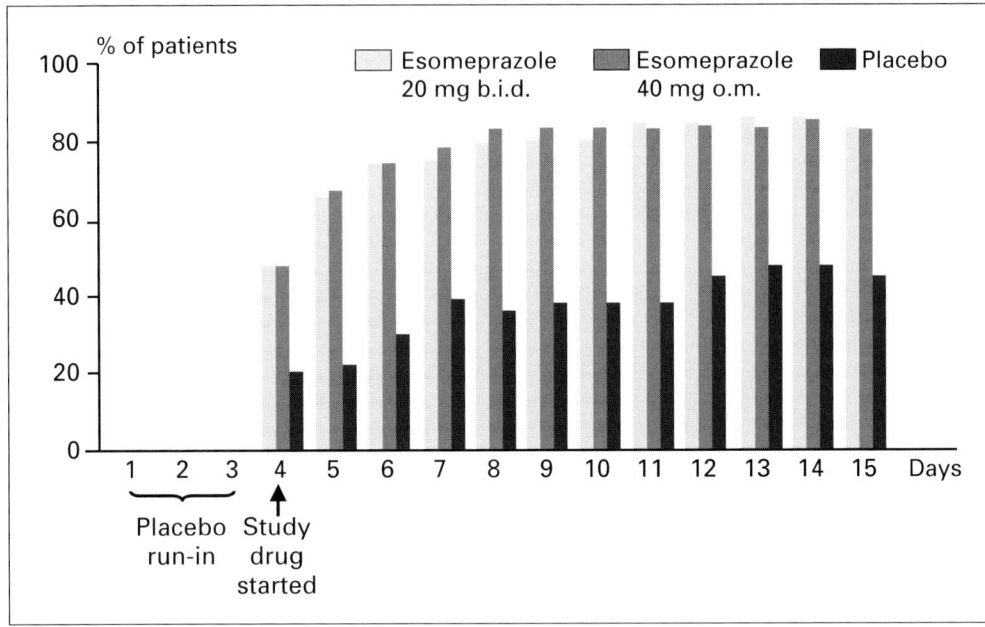

Figure 2. Therapeutic response to PPI as a GERD confirmatory test (modified after [12]).

with documentary differences in the level of acid control over 24 hours between various PPIs. Taken together, it is now apparent that the efficacy of PPIs, to maintain endoscopic healing in the long-term perspective and to relieve GERD patients from their symptoms, are determined by the efficacy by which the drug controls 24-hour intragastric pH.

On demand concept

The primary goals of therapy for the majority of patients with GERD are symptom relief and relapse prevention while healing is also an important outcome for patients with all grades of oesophagitis with or without complications. The choice of therapy for long-term management of GERD should of course always consider the patient's own preferences and opinion. If symptoms are infrequent, then on demand therapy may offer a reasonable approach to management. Indeed in patients who are on regular long-term medication for GERD, it is known that they often only take the drug when symptoms recur. On demand therapy with PPIs may therefore represent a valid option for the long-term management for such patients, particularly since this is probably the method already today used for many patients in clinical practice. Furthermore, the PPI on demand therapy has been shown to be associated with the reduction of antacid usage compared to placebo, and a few patients required treatments for periods of more than three consecutive days. In endoscopy-negative reflux disease 85-90% of patients are willing to continue with on demand PPI therapy [17, 18]. These results suggest that many of similar patients may not require continued maintenance therapy for control of their symptoms. On demand therapy therefore provides a more individualized approach to management of the patients with GERD whereby the patient dictates the extent of the drug usage according to his or her specific needs.

What about *Helicobacter pylori*?

Evaluation of epidemiology data from Western countries describes a negative relationship between the trend for *Helicobacter pylori (Hp)* colonisation and the prevalence of GERD and its long-term complications. This overall trend suggested that the prevalence of *Hp* colonisation is decreasing in Western societies and that the prevalences of GERD and related diseases are rising. Presently there is no direct evidence in favour of the involvement of *Hp* in the pathogenesis of GERD although *Hp* is accepted to have a causal link to peptic ulcer disease. Clinical trial data suggest that the presence of *Hp* has little influence on the effectiveness of anti-secretory efficacy of proton pump inhibitor in patients with *GERD*. A meta-analysis of results from long-term studies suggested that the risk of GERD relapse may be reduced in the presence of *Hp* infection during maintenance treatment. Several investigators have raised concern about increased risk for gastric neoplasia in *Hp* positive patients treated with PPIs. However, long-term follow-up in such patients indicates neither significant risk of neoplasia nor accelerated development of gastric glandular atrophy [19]. However, since *Helicobacter pylori* infection is a crucial factor in the multistep casual pathogenetic process of gastric cancer, there is solid evidence to support the strategy of submitting patients being infected to eradication therapy according to modern principles including triple therapy during one week.

Anti-reflux surgery

Surgical treatment of GERD has previously been limited to patients with chronic complicated reflux and in those with very longstanding, severe symptoms. There is now an increasing tendency in many countries to utilise surgery in earlier stages of the disease [20]. This change in clinical practice is partly due to changes in surgical technique (laparoscopic approach) but it is probably paradoxically also due to the improvement in medical therapy. With the efficacy and availability of modern medical therapy the focus, as well as the opportunities of therapy for GERD, have changed but also the recognition of the magnitude of the impairment in quality of life in patients who are not adequately treated. This increase of the awareness might be the most pregnant cause of the suggested increase of the disease in the adult population. An important background factor for the significant but not eminent strategic decisions to be taken in the long-term management of GERD patients is the fact that there are shortcomings and draw-backs with pharmacological, maintenance therapy. GERD is a disease of chronic nature in which medical therapies are entirely targeting on the control of acid reflux far from correcting the underlying motor abnormalities of the upper alimentary canal. We have to realise that low dose PPI therapy and full dose H_2 receptor antagonists insufficiently interfere with food stimulated acid production and thereby reflux. Profound and sometimes prolonged acid rebound phenomenon is perhaps a greater problem after stopping therapy than previously recognized. Furthermore, in severe reflux disease patients twice daily dosing of the PPI is often necessary. In addition there is sometimes an insufficient control of volume reflux, nocturnal symptoms and retrosternal pain. Acid breakthrough during the night has recently been recognized, the control which requires more complicated management strategies. An additional issue of potential concern is the controversy prevailing regarding the significance of the non-acid reflux components (bile and pancreatic juice constituents) and their probable effects on the occurrence of columnar metaplasia and their impact on the perpetuation of the metaplastic-dysplastic processes leading to the rapidly increasing incidence of adenocarcinoma of the oesophagus [21, 22]. These many concerns have already today an important impact on the attitudes towards complete control of reflux and will definitely have so in the future. Taken together there seems to be a growing demand for the complete and durable control of reflux, based on the principle of reconstruction of the physiology of the gastroesophageal junction, which seems to be a reachable goal when doing a proper anti-reflux operation [23-26].

A number of patient groups can be identified who are particularly suited and recommended to have a laparoscopic anti-reflux operation. This decision is mostly based on the patient's own preferences after a comprehensive and prolonged discussion process with an experienced surgeon. We have a group of patients with complicated reflux disease which is represented by peptic stricture and columnar lined oesophagus; and another group of patients with respiratory complications of reflux in the form of chronic bronchitis, posterior laryngitis and hoarseness. These groups are always difficult to select in order to predict a most favourable outcome after anti-reflux surgery.

Endoscopic treatments for GERD

The ideal situation would be that new therapeutic endoscopic treatments should fulfil certain criteria before they have disseminated into widespread clinical use. The treatment modality requires a physiologic rationale. The technologic procedure should not be too complex or difficult to use. Benefits of the procedure have to outweigh the risks of therapy, *i.e.* it has to be safe with little, or no associated morbidity. Efficacy of therapy should be demonstrated in controlled clinical trials with a sham procedure incorporated. Long-term patient follow-ups should be performed to assess the effects and durability of treatment. The endoscopic treatment should be applicable to the majority of patients with GERD and presumable cost-effective. With the introduction of a spectrum of sophisticated new technologies, most of these requirements have still to be shown. The following devises have reached a quite wide spread use: radiofrequency energy delivered to distal oesophageal tissue (Stretta); suture plication (gastroplasty) involving placing stitches into the proximal gastric folds to form a fundic barrier to prevent reflux; endoscopic implantation of microspheres or polymeres to induce a high pressure barrier to prevent reflux in the lower oesophageal sphincter zone [27, 28]. There is an apparent rush to marketing these new devices before answering many of the questions listed above. These new endoscopic therapies may have a role in the long-term management of GERD but at the moment it would be preferable to only apply these devices only within the framework of controlled randomised clinical trials.

References

1. Spechler SJ. Epidemiology and natural history of gastroesophageal reflux disease. *Digestion* 1992; 51 (Suppl. 1): 24-9.
2. Galmiche JP, Bruley des Varannes S. Symptoms and disease severity in gastroesophageal reflux disease. *Scand J Gastroenterol* 1994; 29 (Suppl. 201): 62-8.
3. Glise H, Hallerbäck B, Johansson B. Quality of life assessments in the evaluation of gastroesophageal reflux and peptic ulcer disease before, during and after treatment. *Scand J Gastroenterol* 1995; 208: 103-35.
4. Dent J, Brun J, Fendrick AM, et al, for the General Workshop Group. An evidence-based appraisal of reflux disease management: the General Workshop Group. *Gut* 1999; 44 (Suppl. 2): S1-16.
5. Lundell L. New information relevant to long-term management of endoscopy-negative reflux disease. *Aliment Pharmacol Ther* 1997; 11 (Suppl. 2): 93-8.
6. Carlsson R, Dent J, Watts R, et al. Gastrooesophageal reflux disease (GORD) in primary care – an international study of different treatment strategies with omeprazole. *Eur J Gastroenterol Hepatol* 1998; 10: 119-24.
7. Schindlebeck NE, Klauser AG, Voderholzer WA, et al. Empiric therapy for gastroesophageal reflux disease. *Arch Intern Med* 1995; 155: 1808-12.
8. Johnsson F, Weyvadt L, Solhaug JH, et al. One-week omeprazole and treatment as a diagnostic test for gastroesophageal reflux disease. *Scand J Gastroenterol* 1998; 33: 15-20.
9. Kamel PL, Hanson D, Kahrilas PJ. Omeprazole for the treatment of posterior laryngitis. *Am J Med* 1994; 96: 321-6.
10. Edwards SJ, Lind T, Lundell L. Review article: systematic review of proton pump inhibitors for the acute treatment of reflux oesophagitis. *Aliment Pharmacol Ther* 2001; 15: 1729-36.
11. Sharma VK, Leonbtiadis GI, Howden CW. Meta-analysis of randomized controlled trials comparing standard clinical doses of omeprazole and lansoprazole in erosive oesophagitis. *Aliment Pharmacol Ther* 2001; 15: 227-31.
12. Johnsson, et al. One-week esomeprazole treatment: an effective confirmatory test in patients with suspected gastroesophageal reflux disease. DDW 2001.
13. Carlsson R, Galmiche JP, Dent J, Lundell L, Frison L. Prognostic factors influencing relapse of oesophagitis during maintenance therapy with antisecretory drugs: a meta-analysis of long-term omeprazole trials. *Aliment Pharmacol Ther* 1997; 11: 472-82.
14. Klinkenberg-Knol EC, Nelis F, Dent J, et al. Long-term omeprazole treatment in resistant gastroesophageal reflux disease: efficacy, safety and influence on gastric mucosa. *Gastroenterology* 2000; 118: 661-9.
15. Lundell L. Acid suppression in the long-term treatment of peptic stricture and Barrett's oesophagus. *Digestion* 1992; 51 (Suppl. 1): 49-58.
16. Marks RD, Richter JE, Rizzo J, et al. Omeprazole vs H_2-receptor antagonists in treating patients with peptic stricture and esophagitis. *Gastroenterology* 1994; 106: 907-15.
17. Lind T, Havelund T, Lundell L, et al. On demand therapy with omeprazole for the long-term management of patients with heartburn without oesophagitis – a placebo-controlled randomized trial. *Aliment Pharmacol Ther* 1999; 13: 907-1014.
18. Talley NJ, Lauritsen K, Tunturi-Hihnalas H, Lind T, Moum B, Bang C, Schultz T, Omland TM, Delle M, Junghard O. Esomeprazole 20 mg maintains symptom control in endoscopy-negative gastroesophageal reflux disease: a controlled trial of "on demand" therapy for six months. *Aliment Pharmacol Ther* 2001; 15: 347-54.
19. Lundell L. Gastro-oesophageal reflux disease in *Helicobacter pylori* or gastroesophageal reflux disease from *Helicobacter pylori*? *Eur J Gastroenterol and Hepatology* 2001; 13 (Suppl. 1): 23-7.
20. Watson DI, Foreman D, Devitt PG, et al. Preoperative endoscopic grading of oesopahgitis vs outcome after laparoscopic Nissen fundoplication. *Am J Gastroenterol* 1997; 92: 222-5.

21. Attwood SE, Smyrk TC, DeMeester TR, et al. Duodenoesophageal reflux and the development of adenocarcinoma in rats. *Surgery* 1992; 111: 503-10.
22. Lagergren J, Bergström R, Lindgren A, et al. Symptomatic gastroesophageal reflux as a risk factor for esopahgeal adenocarcinoma. *N Engl Med* 1999; 18: 340: 825-31.
23. Ortiz A, Martinez LF, Parrilla P, et al. Conservative treatment *vs* antireflux surgery in Barrett's oesophagus: long-term results of a prospective study. *Br J Surg* 1996; 83: 274-8.
24. Csendes A, Braghetto I, Burdiles P, et al. Long-term results of classic antireflux surgery in 152 patients with Barrett's esophagus: clinical radiologic, endoscopic, manometric and acid reflux test analysis before and late after operation. *Surg* 1998; 123: 645-57.
25. Rydberg L, Ruth M, Lundell L. Does oesophageal motor function improve with time after successful antireflux surgery? Results of a prospective, randomised clinical study. *Gut* 1997; 41: 82-6.
26. Lundell L, Abrahamsson H, Ruth M, et al. Long-term results of a prospective randomised comparison of total fundic wrap (Nissen-Rossetti) or semifundoplication (Toupet) for gastroesophageal reflux. *Br J Surg* 1996; 83: 830-35.
27. Filipi CJ, Lehman GA, Rothstein RI, et al. Transoral flexible endoscopic suturing for treatment of gastroesophageal reflux disease: a multicenter trial. *Gastrointest Endosc* 2001; 53: 416-26.
28. Triadafilopoulous G, Baise JK, Nostrant TT, et al. Radio frequency energy delivery to the gastroesophageal function for the treatment of gastroesophageal reflux disease. *Gastrointest Endosc* 2001; 53: 407-15.

New insights in the molecular etiopathogenesis of inflammatory bowel disease

Jürgen Schölmerich

Department of Internal Medicine I, University Medical Center Regensburg, Regensburg, Germany

Abstract

It is meanwhile generally accepted that susceptibility genes and environmental factors are of importance regarding etiology of inflammatory bowel diseases. It is obvious that susceptibility genes are located on different chromosomes. Thus far, however, only the NOD-2 mutation which probably leads to a disturbed interaction of luminal bacteria with the mucosa associated immune system has been defined. This mutation is responsible for 10-20% of patients with Crohn's disease. It remains to be seen what functions other susceptibility genes will have. Environmental factors include bacterial flora, nutritional components, drugs, toxins and probably childhood hygiene or factors associated with higher social standard. It is clear that subgroups of both, Crohn's disease and ulcerative colitis, will exist having different phenotypes as well as different genotypes.
A vast number of mediators is involved in pathophysiology. The system seems to be very much redundant and therefore difficult to modulate. A dysfunstion of epithelial cells and the epithelial barrier may be the clue to both, etiology and pathophysiology. The detection of further gene mutations will hopefully lead to a much clearer picture and finally to reasonable treatments. Alternatives to the immunological paradigm may also exist and need to be studied.

Although the chronic inflammatory bowel diseases (IBD) are meanwhile more than 100 years old, their etiology and pathophysiology is still not really clarified. However, in the last two decades many findings regarding genetics, patient phenotypes, environmental influences, abnormal immune reaction, inflammatory signals and signal transduction have been brought forward, and the mosaic starts to become understandable. In the following short review only a few points can be discussed focussing on genetic susceptibility, patients subgrouping, environmental influence on manifestation and in particular bacterial epithelial interactions, cytokines and finally alternative hypotheses. An understanding of etiology and thereby causal therapy or prevention would obviously be the optimal way to develop definitive treatments not yet found in spite of intensive research and development.

The example of the cotton-top tamarin *(Saguinus oedipus oedipus)* which lives in the wild in Central America and has rarely (as far as it is known) chronic IBD gives a paradigm for the human diseases. If kept in captivity, these animals develop chronic IBD which very much resemble those of man. They have a familiar concordance if monkey families are analyzed, which points to a genetic background. The manifestation of the disease only after transfer into captivity shows in addition the influence of environmental factors. Since the animals show three different types of diseases, we also learn that subgroups of IBD must exist.

Genetics

The most important argument for a existence of a genetic susceptibility came from twin studies showing that monozygote twins have a concordance rate which is significantly higher than those in heterozygote twins which have only 50% identity [1]. Numerous studies on familiar aggregation of IBD point into the same direction.

However, the functional substrate of genetic susceptibility is thus far still elusive. The search for the responsible genes followed the "Casablanca method": arrest the usual suspects. Cytokines, cytokine ratios and many other known abnormal parameters were studied regarding their genetic background without much positive results. For example the ratio of pro- and anti-inflammatory cytokines, in particular interleukin-1 and its endogenous receptor antagonist has been proposed as a genetic abnormality but this has not been confirmed using appropriate controls [2, 3]. Increased permeability has been demonstrated in early studies of Hollander in patients and in relatives of patients with Crohn's disease [4]. These findings have been reproduced by others but not by all authors. Thus, a barrier defect is considered as a possible causal factor.

The search for the genes finally led to numerous chromosomal locations of susceptibility loci although only a smaller number of findings has been coroborated by independent studies. Recently the first IBD gene was found which if mutated seems to be responsible for 10% to 20% of patients with Crohn's disease in Caucasians *(Figure 1)* [5-7]. The mutation seems to be associated in particular with ileal involvement [8], it is at least more frequent with ileal as compared to colonic involvement (26.9% *versus* 12.7%) [9]. It also seems to be more frequently associated with the stricturing phenotype (53% *versus* 28%) [10]. It is still unclear how the NOD-2 mutation allows for the manifestation of Crohn's disease. Abnormal interaction of bacteria or bacterial products with the NFκB signaling cascade may be one explanation *(Figure 1)*.

The fact that this mutation accounts for a subgroup of patients with Crohn's disease and that it seems to be associated with specific location and maybe behavior points to different phenotypes or subgroups in IBD *(see below)*. For ulcerative colitis thus far no major breakthrough regarding the description of a genetic abnormality has been made. There are some data supporting the more frequent occurrence of a polymorphism for multiple

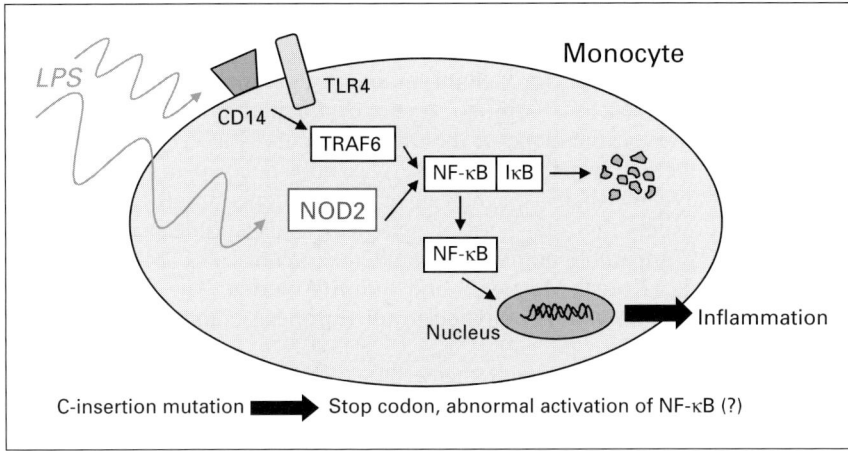

Figure 1. Identification of the first IBD-gene – NOD2.

drug resistance protein 1 (MDR-1) which is associated with a lower expression of this protein [11] but this remains to be reproduced. Interestingly in a mouse model knockout of this gene led to colitis as well [12]. The abnormal expression of MDR-1 could explain abnormal export of bacterial products or toxins from epithelial cells and thereby an influence on chronic inflammation.

Patient subgroups

The high number of chromosomal locations, the fact that a known mutation covers only a subset of patients and daily clinical experience with very different types of patients and disease phenotypes point to the fact that Crohn's disease and probably ulcerative colitis as well do not represent a single entity but the expression of quite different primary defects with a limited array of expression in the intestinal tract. It is obvious that a patient with a short fibrosing change of the ileocoecal junction is different from a patient with extensive fistulizing and perforating abnormalities in the rectal area or even involvement of the oral cavity or the upper GI tract. There are data from the surgical and from the medical literature providing evidence that the different types regarding location and behavior are correlated with a different relapse risk, a different time to relapse and a different response to drugs. The recently published Vienna Classification which has been worked out by an international group [13] provides one attempt for a patient classification in Crohn's disease. This needs, however, to be refined and possibly serological markers may be helpful as well (*i.e.* pANCA or ASCA).

Environmental factors

Epidemiological studies show a North-South gradient regarding the incidence of Crohn's disease in Europe and therefore point to an environmental factor earlier occurring in Northern Europe. However, the slope of the incidence curves is very similar in Northern as compared to Southern Europe, the increase was only delayed in time from North to South. As far as analyzable there is a plateau of the incidence in all European countries which probably represents the total pool of genetically susceptible people. Interestingly during the last years comparable numbers of incidence increases have been found in some countries in East Asia (Korea, Malaysia) and South America. The incidence increases, however, are delayed again when compared to all European countries.

The search for a given environmental factor able to induce abnormal reactions of the mucosal immune system based on a genetic susceptibility has led to an abundance of proposals including food preservatives, a number of ingredients of westernized food and others. One possible factor is hygiene in early childhood. Epidemiological studies from the United Kingdom have pointed out that the availability of a hot water tap or a separate toilet in early childhood is associated with a significant increased risk of a manifestation of Crohn's disease in later life [14] *(Table I)*. Thus, a limited hygiene in early childhood would be a protective factor. These findings have been reproduced by others and are in accordance with data showing that the presence of older siblings in families which bring infections from kindergarten or school to the younger siblings protects against later occurrence of Crohn's disease as well.

Other factors which are compatible with the epidemiology of the disease are for example the frequent application of drugs such as non-steroidal anti-inflammatory drugs or antibiotics in the westernized countries which may also be responsible for the manifestation of the disease if genetic susceptibility is present.

Table I. Hygiene in childhood-IBD. (From [14])

	RR	
	CD	UC
Hot water tap	5.0 (1.4 - 17.3)	1.3 (0.7 - 2.2)
Water tap	1.8 (0.6 - 5.4)	0.9 (0.5 - 1.7)
Separate toilet	3.3 (1.3 - 8.3)	1.3 (0.7 - 2.4)
Canalisation	2.6 (0.9 - 7.3)	1.2 (0.7 - 2.1)
Appendectomy	1.4 (0.6 - 3.4)	0.3 (0.1 - 0.6)

Bacterial epithelial interactions

In health the 10^{14} bacteria in the gut have a well-balanced interaction with the huge surface of the intestinal tract. Although the bacteria outnumber the human cells and probably their different genes outnumber the human genes and maybe even human proteins, there is a homeostasis which is rarely disturbed *(Figure 2)*. Bacteria have a significant influence on the expression of the genes in the intestinal cells [15] *(Table II)*. They also have an

Table II. Influence of colonisation on gene expression in the intestine. (From [15])

	Increase (xfold)*
Na$^+$/glucose cotransporter	2.6 ± 0.9
Colipase	6.6 ± 1.9
Metallothionein	- 5.4 ± 0.7
Immunoglobulin receptor	2.6 ± 0.7
Multidrug resistance protein (Mdr 1a)	- 3.8 ± 1.0
Small proline rich protein 2a	205 ± 64

* Relative to germfree.

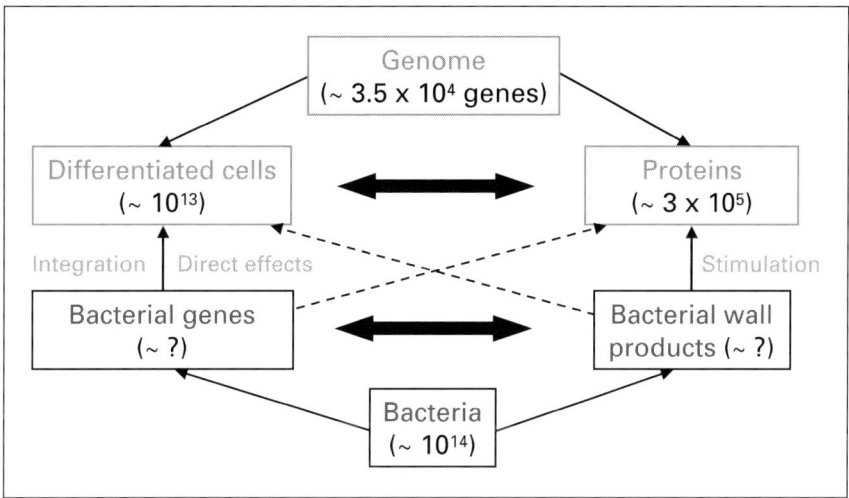

Figure 2. Components of the human organism.

important influence on intestinal permeability which depends on the species studied – some bacteria increase and some decrease permeability as measured by mannitol clearance [16] *(Figure 3)*. Numerous studies point to the importance of the endogenous flora for the manifestation and the perpetuation of intestinal inflammation in susceptible hosts [17]. Practically all animal models thus far described are dependent on the presence of bacteria as shown for example for the colitis in interleukin-2 knock-out mice [18] *(Figure 4)*. The fact that genetically engineered bacteria secreting interleukin-10 have positive effects on two different models of intestinal inflammation [19] and that in addition, the application of cytosine-guanosine-motifs of bacterial DNA have a preventive effect for several models of experimental colitis [20] underline the importance of bacteria for the manifestation and maybe for the later treatment of inflammatory bowel disorders. In particular the fact that the tolerance toward resident intestinal flora is broken in active IBD [21] *(Table III)* demonstrates that this is also true for humans.

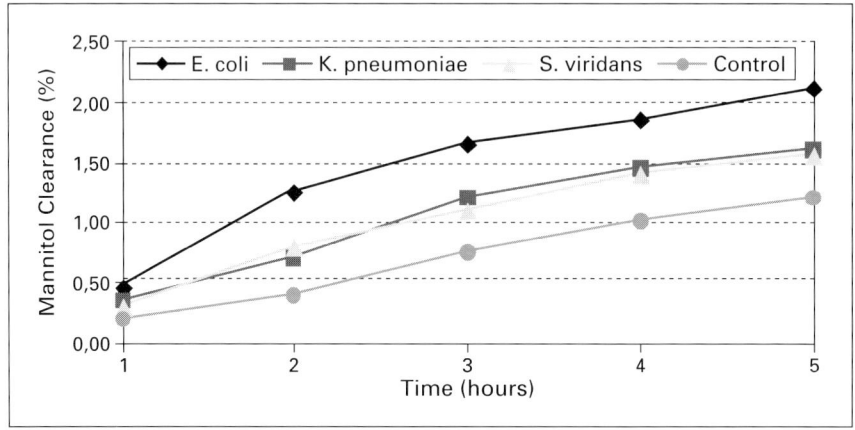

Figure 3. Bacteria and intestinal permeability. (From [16].)

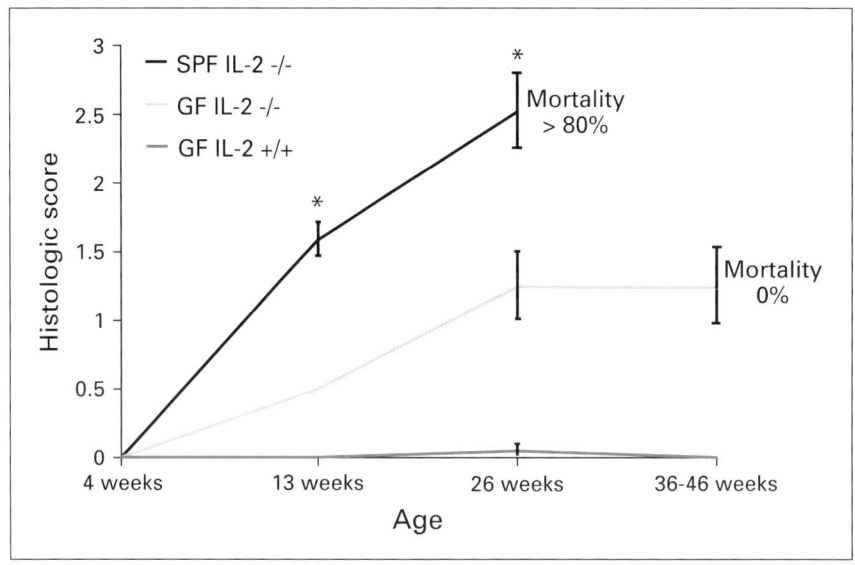

Figure 4. Colitis in IL-2 knockout mice. (From [18].) * p < 0.0001.

Table III. Tolerance towards resident intestinal flora is broken in active IBD. (From [21])

	BSA		BSH	
	Anaerob	Aerob	Anaerob	Aerob
Controls (n = 9/6)	751*	710	11756	12276
CD inactive (n = 6/3)	698	800	8719	12462
CD active (n = 5/3)	17553	15467	8109	8410

* Proliferation as ct/min.
Tolerance can be restored (in mice) by IL-10 or anti-IL-12!
BS: bacterial sonicate; A: autologous; H: heterologous.

Other potential defects

Defective apoptosis of intestinal immune cells may be an important determinant for another subgroup of patients. It could well be that these are the patients which are responsive to treatment with apoptosis-inducing agents such as infliximab and others [22, 23].

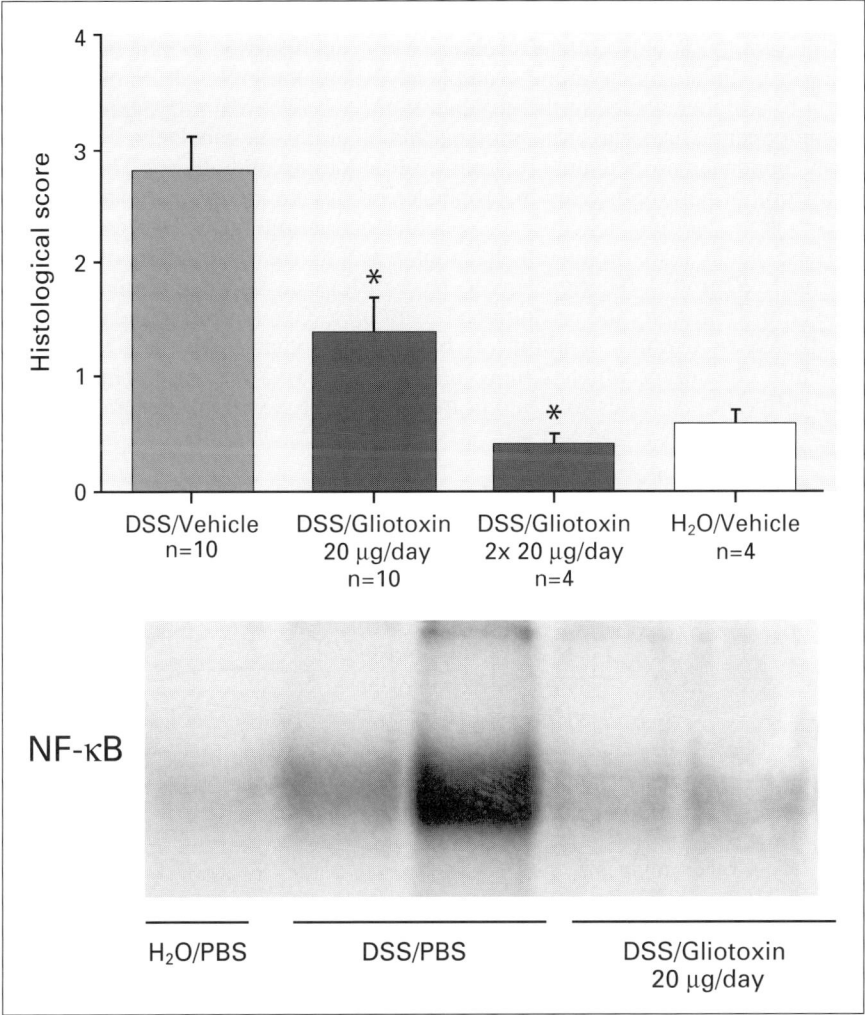

Figure 5. Gliotoxin suppresses acute DSS-induced colitis and inhibits NFκB binding activity *in vivo*. (From [28].)

Cytokines and signal transduction

Although no real evidence has been found for primarily disturbed cytokine production or synthesis, it is generally accepted that several cytokines are involved in the pathophysiology of intestinal inflammation in IBD. The same is true for the major nuclear transcription factor NFκB [24]. Experiments blocking different cytokines have shown that they are important for the perpetuation of chronic inflammation but on the other hand that there is redundancy which makes it difficult to influence abnormalities or even disease blocking only one of them [25]. It is also known that blockade of the nuclear translocation of NFκB ameliorates or prevents experimental colitis and in a few patients the human disease as well [26-29] *(Figure 5)*.

While etiology remains still somehow elusive, most experts agree on the major pathways on pathophysiology. It is for obvious reasons very much related to general inflammation which has been studied again on the example of IBD on a high level. Immune cells which are present to a higher degree in the gut than in the whole remaining organism react with luminal components (bacteria, virus, proteins and others) in an unbalanced way and release thereby an abundance of mediators (cytokines, chemokines and others). These in turn lead to the attraction of neutrophils and macrophages producing again an abundance of further mediators (prostaglandins, leucotrienes, platelet activating factor, oxygen radicals and more). These again lead finally on different ways to the destruction of the intestinal epithelial cell *(Figure 6)*. There seems to be a difference between Crohn's disease and ulcerative colitis regarding the predominant cytokines. This has led to the impression that Crohn's disease or Crohn's syndrome is basically associated with a T-helper cell response 1 while ulcerative colitis is more related to a TH-2 response. This may explain somewhat different responses to different treatments but is still not generally accepted as

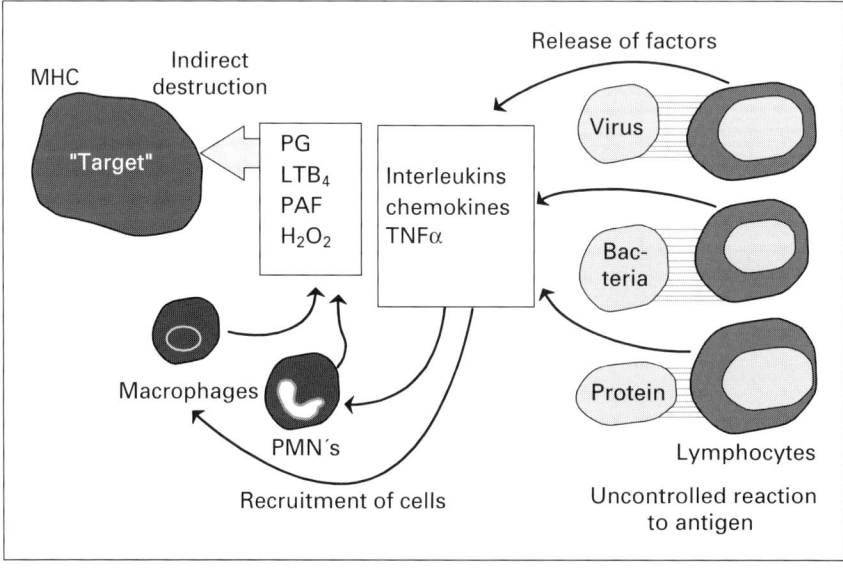

Figure 6. Principles of pathophysiology of IBD.

initial principle. This scheme *(Figure 6)* provides the rationale why all drugs used thus far with success have a pluripotent character meaning that they inhibit as a rule a relatively high number of mediators or their production. This is true for 5-ASA as well as for steroids and conventional immunosuppressives. The comparison of this plethora of mediators with an orchestra clarifies that the inhibition of a single mediator is probably as ineffective as a deletion of a single instrument from the orchestra [30]. The fact that most of the recently developed "anti-cytokine" or "anti-adhesion" treatments have been of very little efficacy [31] indicates that the inflammatory system in the intestinal mucosa has a high redundancy which makes it unlikely that the inhibition of single mediators is really a rational approach *(Table IV)*.

Table IV. "Biological treatments" for IBD. State of development 10/2002

Substance	CD	UC
IL-1 RA	(-)	?
TNF-AK	+	(+)
RNF-R 75 und 55	-	?
MAP-kinase-inhibitor	?	?
NFκB p65 antisense	(+)	(+)
Anti-CD4	+	?
Anti-IL-12	(-)	?
Anti-INFγ	-	?
Anti-Il-2 R	(+)	?
IL-10	(+)	?
Anti-α4 integrin	(+)	?
Anti-α4β7 integrin	?	(-)
Anti-ICAM-1	-	?
EGF	?	(?)
KGF	?	-
INFα	(-)	(-)
INFβ	(-)	(+)
GCSF/GMCSF	(+)	?
Growth hormone	(+)	?
DHEA	(+)	(+)
IL-11	(-)	?

Alternative concepts

The failure of most of the recently developed biological therapies may also indicate that the basic paradigm of a primary immunological abnormality is wrong. Although it is obvious that bacterial epithelial interactions play a significant role in manifestation and probably in perpetuation of intestinal inflammation, the causes of this disturbed interaction can be of non-immunological basis and may even be localized in distant organs such as the liver. A number of hypotheses have been brought forward, for example suggesting that effects in xenobiotic metabolism in the liver due to a genetic abnormality of metabolizing enzymes [32] or as indicated above ABC transporters may be the underlying problem for a subset of patients. The description of the MDR-1 polymorphism *(Table V)* may be indicative of one such example. The fact that in some animal models the application of hydrophilic bile acids improves experimental ileitis and colitis points into the same direction *(Table VI)* [33, 34].

Table V. MDR-1 polymorphism in IBD. (From [11])

C 3435 T-substitution: P-glycoprotein ↓

	CC	CT	TT
UC (n = 149)	17 (12 - 25)*	52 (43 - 60)	31 (24 - 39)
Control	26 (19 - 34)	51 (43 - 59)	23 (16 - 30)
CD (n = 129)	26 (18 - 35)	54 (45 - 63)	20 (13 - 28)
Control	28 (20 - 36)	46 (37 - 55)	26 (19 - 35)

* % (95% CI).
UC *vs* Control $p < 0.045$.

Table VI. UDCA improves experimental ileitis and colitis.
(From [33, 34])

	Macroscopic score	
	Vehicle	URSO
Indomethacin-ileitis	6.2 ± 1.4	3.0 ± 2.5*
TNB-colitis	3.6 ± 1.4	1.8 ± 1.6*

* $p < 0.05$.
Microscopic score, MPO, weight were also favourably influenced.

Summary

Thus far it is clear that genetics and environmental factors are important for etiology. No specific genetic determinant has yet been found except for the NOD-2 mutation where the functional defect is not completely clear. Increased permeability, abnormal cytokine function and many other suggestions are abundant. Environmental factors include bacterial flora, nutritional components, drugs, toxins and probably childhood hygiene or factors associated with a higher social standard. Probably several genes and several environmental factors are involved in different subgroups. A vast number of mediators is involved in pathophysiology. The system seems to be very much redundant and therefore difficult to modulate. A dysfunction of epithelial cells and the epithelial barrier might be the clue to both – etiology and pathophysiology. Detection of further genes may lead to a much clearer picture and finally to reasonable treatments. Alternatives to the immunological paradigm need to be studied even if of little interest to drug development companies.

References

1. Tysk C, Lindberg E, Jarnerot G, Floderus-Myrhed B. Ulcerative colitis and Crohn's disease in an unselected population of monozygotic and dizygotic twins. A study of heritability and the influence of smoking. *Gut* 1988; 29: 990-6.
2. Casini-Raggi V, Kam L, Chong YJ, Fiocchi C, Pizarro TT, Cominelli F. Mucosal imbalance of IL-1 and IL-1 receptor antagonist in inflammatory bowel disease. A novel mechanism of chronic intestinal inflammation. *J Immunol* 1995; 154: 2434-40.
3. Andus T, Daig R, Vogl D, Aschenbrenner E, Lock G, Hollerbach S, Köllinger M, Schölmerich J, Gross V. Imbalance of the interleukin-1 system in colonic mucosa-association with intestinal inflammation and interleukin-1 receptor antagonist genotype 2. *Gut* 1997; 41: 651-7.
4. Hollander D, Vadheim CM, Brettholz E, Petersen GM, Delahunty T, Rotter JI. Increased intestinal permeability in patients with Crohn's disease and their relatives. A possible etiologic factor. *Ann Intern Med* 1986; 105: 883-5.
5. Ogura Y, Bonen DK, Inohara N, Nicolae DL, Chen FF, Ramos R, Britton H, Moran T, Karaliuskas R, Duerr RH, Achkar JP, Brant SR, Bayless TM, Kirschner BS, Hanauer SB, Nunez G, Cho JH. A frameshift mutation in NOD2 associated with susceptibility to Crohn's disease. *Nature* 2001; 411: 603-6.
6. Hugot JP, Chamaillard M, Zouali H, Lesage S, Cezard JP, Belaiche J, Almer S, Tysk C, O'Morain CA, Gassull M, Binder V, Finkel Y, Cortot A, Modigliani R, Laurent-Puig P, Gower-Rousseau C, Macry J, Colombel JF, Sahbatou M, Thomas G. Association of NOD2 leucine-rich repeat variants with susceptibility to Crohn's disease. *Nature* 2001; 411: 599-603.
7. Hampe J, Cuthbert A, Croucher PJP, Mirza MM, Mascheretti S, Fisher S, Frenzel H, King K, Hasselmeyer A, MacPherson AJS, Bridger S, van Deventer S, Forbes A, Nikolaus S, Lennard-Jones JE, Foelsch UR, Krawczak M, Lewis C, Schreiber S, Mathew CG. Association between insertion mutation in NOD2 gene and Crohn's disease in German and British populations. *Lancet* 2001; 357: 1925-8.
8. Ahmad T, Armuzzi A, Bunce M, Mulcahy-Hawes K, Marshall SE, Orchard TR, Crawshaw J, Large O, de Silva A, Cook JT, Barnardo M, Cullen S, Welsh KI, Jewell DP. The molecular classification of the clinical manifestations of Crohn's disease. *Gastroenterology* 2002; 122: 854-66.
9. Cuthbert AP, Fisher SA, Mirza MM, King K, Hampe J, Croucher PJ, Mascheretti S, Sanderson J, Forbes A, Mansfield J, Schreiber S, Lewis CM, Mathew CG. The contribution of NOD2 gene mutations to the risk and site of disease in inflammation bowel disease. *Gastroenterology* 2002; 122: 867-74.
10. Lesage S, Zouali H, Cezard JP, Colombel JF, Belaiche J, Almer S, Tysk C, O'Morain C, Gassull M, Binder V, Finkel Y, Modigliani R, Gower-Rousseau C, Macry J, Merlin F, Chamaillard M, Jannot AS, Thomas G, Hugot JP; EPWG-IBD Group; EPIMAD Group; GETAID Group. CARD15/NOD2 mutational analysis and genotype-phenotype correlation in 612 patients with inflammatory bowel disease. *Am J Hum Genet* 2002; 70: 845-57.
11. Schwab M, Schaeffler E, Fromm M, Marx C, Metzler J, Stange E, Herfarth H, Schoelmerich J, Kaskas B, Gregor M, Walker S, Cascorbi I, Roots I, Brinkmann U, Zanger UM, Eichelbaum M. Contribution of the C 3435 T MDR 1 gene polymorphism for susceptibility in inflammatory bowel disease. Submitted.
12. Panwala CM, Jones JC, Viney JL. A novel model of inflammatory bowel disease: mice deficient for the multiple drug resistance gene, mdr1a, spontaneously develop colitis. *J Immunol* 1998; 161: 5733-44.
13. Gasché C, Schölmerich J, Brynskow J, D'Haens G, Hanauer SB, Irvine EJ, Jewell DP, Rachmilewitz D, Sachar DB, Sandborn WJ, Sutherland LR. A simple classification of Crohn's disease: report of the Working Party for the World Congresses of Gastroenterology, Vienna 1998. *Inflamm Bowel Dis* 2000; 6: 8-15.

14. Gent AE, Hellier MD, Grace RH, Swarbrick ET, Coggon D. Inflammatory bowel disease and domestic hygiene in infancy. *Lancet* 1994; 343: 766-7.
15. Hooper LV, Wong MH, Thelin A, Hansson L, Falk PG, Gordon JI. Molecular analysis of commensal host-microbial relationships in the intestine. *Science* 2001; 29: 881-4.
16. Garcia-Lafuente A, Antolin M, Guarner F, Crespo E, Malagelada JR. Modulation of colonic barrier function by the composition of the commensal flora in the rat. *Gut* 2001; 48: 503-7.
17. Elson CO. Genes, microbes, and T cells – new therapeutic targets in Crohn's disease. *N Engl J Med* 2002; 346: 614-6.
18. Schultz M, Tonkonogy SL, Sellon RK, Veltkamp C, Godfrey VL, Kwon J, Grenther WB, Balish E, Horak I, Sartor RB. IL-2-deficient mice raised under germfree conditions develop delayed mild focal intestinal inflammation. *Am J Physiol* 1999; 276: G1461-72.
19. Steidler L, Hans W, Schotte L, Neirynck S, Obermeier F, Falk W, Fiers W, Remaut E. Treatment of murine colitis by *Lactococcus lactis* secreting interleukin-10. *Science* 2000; 289: 1352-5.
20. Obermeier F, Dunger N, Deml L, Herfarth H, Schölmerich J, Falk W. CpG motifs of bacterial DNA exacerbate colitis of dextran sulfate sodium-treated mice. *Eur J Immunol* 2002; 32: 2084-92.
21. Duchmann R, Neurath MF, Meyer zum Büschenfelde KH. Responses to self and non-self intestinal microflora in health and inflammatory bowel disease. *Res Immunol* 1997; 148: 589-94.
22. Ina K, Itoh J, Fukushima K, Kusugami K, Yamaguchi T, Kyokane K, Imada A, Binion DG, Musso A, West GA, Dobrea GM, McCormick TS, Lapetina EG, Levine AD, Ottaway CA, Fiocchi C. Resistance of Crohn's disease T cells to multiple apoptotic signals is associated with a Bcl-2/Bax mucosal imbalance. *J Immunol* 1999; 163: 1081-90.
23. Beutler B. Autoimmunity and apoptosis: the Crohn's connection. *Immunity* 2001; 15: 5-14.
24. Rogler G, Brand K, Vogel D, Page S, Hofmeiseter R, Andus T, Knüchel R, Bäuerle PA, Schölmerich J, Gross V. Nuclear factor κB is activated in macrophages and epithelial cells of inflamed intestinal mucosa. *Gastroenterology* 1998; 115: 357-69.
25. Kojouharoff G, Hans W, Obermeier F, Männel DN, Andus T, Schölmerich J, Gross V, Falk W. Neutralization of tumour necrosis factor (TNF) but not of IL-1 reduces inflammation in chronic dextran sulphate sodium-induced colitis in mice. *Clin Exp Immunol* 1997; 107: 353-8.
26. Neurath MF, Pettersson S, Meyer zum Büschenfelde KH, Strober W. Local administration of antisense phosporothioate oligonucleotides to the p65 subunit of NF-B abrogates established experimental colitis in mice. *Nat Med* 1996; 2: 998-1004.
27. Conner EM, Brand S, Davis JM, Laroux FS, Palombella VJ, Fuseler JW, Kang DY, Wolf RE, Grisham MB. Proteasome inhibition attenuates nitric oxide synthase expression, VCAM-1 transcription and the development of chronic colitis. *J Pharmacol Exp Ther* 1997; 282: 1615-22.
28. Herfarth H, Brand K, Rath HC, Rogler G, Schölmerich J, Falk W. Nuclear factor-kappa B activity and intestinal inflammation in dextran sulphate sodium (DSS)-induced colitis in mice is suppressed by gliotoxin. *Clin Exp Immunol* 2000; 120: 59-65.
29. Loefberg R, Neurath M, Ost A, Pettersson S. Topical NFκB p65 antisense oligonucleotides in patients with active distal colonic IBD. A randomised, controlled pilot trial. *Gastroenterology* 2002; 122: A60.
30. Schölmerich J. Future developments in diagnosis and treatment of inflammatory bowel disease. *Hepato-Gastroenterology* 2000; 47: 100-14.
31. Sandborn WJ, Targan SR. Biologic therapy of inflammatory bowel disease. *Gastroenterology* 2002; 122: 1592-1608.
32. Crotty B. Ulcerative colitis and xenobiotic metabolism. *Lancet* 1994; 343: 35-8.
33. Kullmann F, Arndt H, Gross V, Rüschoff J, Schölmerich J. Beneficial effect of ursodeoxycholic acid on mucosal damage in trinitrobenzene sulphonic acid-induced colitis. *Eur J Gastroenterol Hepatol* 1997; 9: 1205-11.
34. Kullmann F, Gross V, Rüschoff J, Arndt H, Benda W, Winkler von Mohrenfels A, Schölmerich J. Effect of ursodeoxycholic acid on the inflammatory activity of indomethacin-induced intestinal inflammation in rats. *Z Gastroenterol* 1997; 35: 171-8.

Drug development based on the molecular mechanisms and current strategies for therapy of inflammatory bowel disease

Stefan Schreiber

Ist Medical Department, Christian-Albrechts-University Kiel, Germany

Abstract

Inflammatory bowel disease (IBD) now serves as a model for modern drug development. The clear phenotype, which appears to allow the definition of "hard" outcome parameters such as mucosal inflammation by endoscopy, has attracted clinical trials with new therapeutic principles. Clinical trials of novel drugs for registration as a treatment for IBD are often pursued on a "proof-of-principle" basis in the development strategy of companies that aim for larger markets in other chronic inflammatory conditions (e.g. rheumatoid arthritis, psoriasis). Drug companies are attracted by the successful development story of the first anti-TNF agent, which has been followed as a paradigm for the development of other experimental drugs. With only two phase II-III multicenter trials, registration needs were satisfied for infliximab for Crohn's disease. Approval for rheumatoid arthritis could be achieved with one additional large, placebo-controlled trial. With the advent of oral drugs that target inflammatory molecules previously identified as effective targets by biologicals, drug development strategies will return to the traditionally structured schemes of three development phases (phase I – toxicity, phase II – dose ranging and definition of application schedule, phase III – clinical efficacy and side effects).

Available pathophysiology-based targeted therapies: TNF-binding agents

The development of TNF neutralizing drugs may serve as a showcase for the application of pathophysiologic insights into actual therapy. It should be pointed out that many other pathophysiology-based therapeutic principles with similar prospects of efficacy are under current development.

Pathophysiological role of TNF

Enhanced secretion of TNF plays an important role in the pathophysiology of IBD [1-3]. TNF induces activation of nuclear factor kappa B (NFkB) amongst other signaling events. Activation of NFkB, which is strongly observed in Crohn's disease [4-6] contributes to many of the destructive cellular and functional events observed in IBD, which are induced or regulated by TNF. Genetic variants in the promoter of the TNF gene or in the TNF molecule itself are not involved as primary factors in the etiology of IBD [7]. However, certain single nucleotide polymorphisms in the TNF promoter induce an increase in TNF-expression [8], which could result in an increased severity factor in Crohn's disease. From its central role in pathophysiology it appears likely that the majority of disease genes that will subsequently be unveiled as important in IBD could be involved in the regulation of TNF or TNF related processes. For example, the recent discovery of the first major disease for Crohn's disease, NOD2 [26-28], suggests that an altered regulation of NFkB activation (and hence activation of TNF) plays an important role in NOD2 related pathophysiology [9].

Therapeutic efficacy

The clinical efficacy of the first targeted approach to IBD was exciting news in 1995: the successful design and presumed efficacy of a drug, infliximab, to specifically inhibit an immunologic mediator, TNF α, was quite exciting in the field, when compared to the broad drug discovery strategies employed in the past [10]. Infliximab is an IgG1 molecule of murine descent that is directed against human TNF and which has been chimerized by replacement of large parts of the antibody's signaling sequence with human DNA sequence. For the first time in IBD therapy, a drug was successfully engineered all the way from the laboratory bench to the bedside. The neutralisation of TNF by parenteral administration of infliximab leads to a vast improvement in some but not all patients with Crohn's disease [11-14]. Through repeated administration of infliximab, a subset of patients with Crohn's disease can be maintained in remission [14] and their fistula apparently remain closed [15] if therapy is continued over a one-year period. Efficacy of infliximab in ulcerative colitis is unclear. A first randomised, controlled clinical trial could not generate a positive signal [16].

Potential differences between TNF-binding drugs

Most interestingly, different agents that neutralize TNF through binding appear to convey different clinical efficacies in Crohn's disease. Etanercept (a fusion protein between TNF-receptor II and an immunoglobulin) has not shown any statistically significant clinical efficacy in comparison with placebo in a small trial [17]. The clinical development of humicade (CDP571, a humanized mouse monoclonal against TNF, that is of IgG1 subclass) appears to run into problems, although therapeutic efficacy has been demonstrated in comparison with placebo [18]. Results of the clinical exploration of TBP-1 (recombinant soluble TNF-receptor I) and CDP870 (polyethylene glycol conjugated ("PEGylated") F(ab')2 fragments directed against TNF) are expected from ongoing clinical trials, with positive signals that have been already observed in small studies. Adalizumab (D2E7, a completely human monoclonal antibody directed against TNF (developed using phage-display technology) is just entering clinical trials in Crohn's disease, but is expected to receive approval for therapy of rheumatoid arthritis within the next year.

Anti-TNF compounds may differ in their biological actions, thus resulting in different levels of clinical efficacy. Differentiating factors could include the ability to induce reverse signaling through binding of membrane expressed TNF [19, 20] as well as cytotoxic or pro-apoptotic capabilities [21-23].

Interindividual differences in drug response. Pharmacogenetic aspects?

There is significant diversity in drug response to anti-TNF drugs in the patient population [11, 12]. Four weeks after a single infusion of infliximab (5 mg/kg bodyweight), about 30-40% of patients are in complete remission, while in others, an incomplete response or no effect is seen. A repeated infusion of 5 mg/kg body weight within 2 weeks induces response (drop of CDAI by at least 70 points) in an additional 13% of patients [14]. It appears that non-responsiveness in not a general phenomenon but rather the result of a differential ability of the TNF-binding antibody to modulate the underlying disease process [12]. While remission rates are very high one week after treatment with a single infusion of infliximab, this effect declines with time [12] leaving only a few patients (up to 13% one year after single infusion) as long-term responders [14]. Immunologic studies suggest that the underlying disease process rebounds, with reactivation of TNF expression and NFkB activation [12].

The variability of response amongst patients and the stability of the pattern after re-exposure appear to be good starting point for pharmacogenetic exploration. Genetic makers would be highly useful as part of the therapeutic algorithm if one could select patients who have a particularly high chance for induction of remission or are at a particular risk for certain side-effects before administration of the drug *(Figure 1)*. Two cohorts from

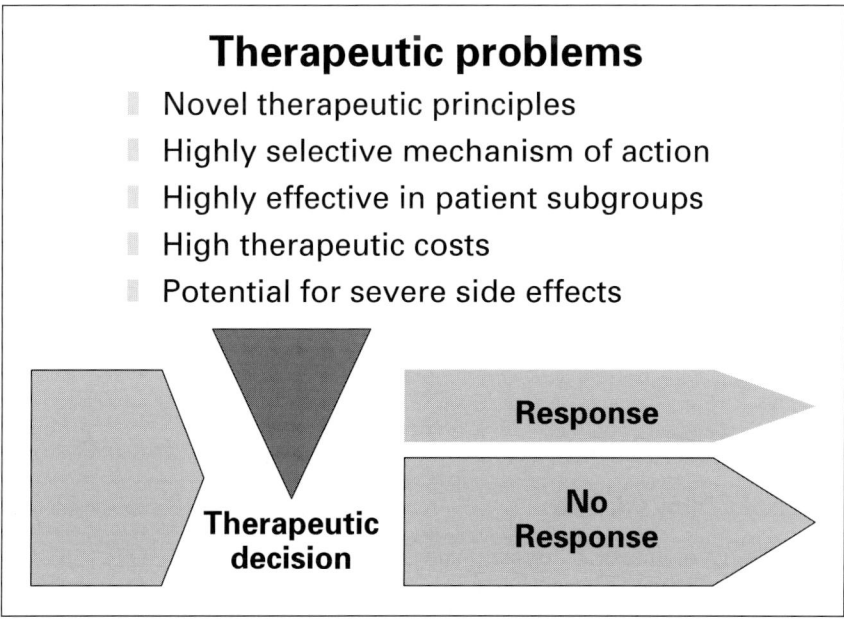

Figure 1. Therapeutic decisions in biologic therapies in inflammatory bowel disease.

multicenter, placebo-controlled trials have been investigated. The combination of the two cohorts results in a high specificity and an adequate power to reject negative findings. In a first series of experiments genetic variation in the TNF-gene itself and the TNF-receptor (I and II) genes could be excluded as pharmacogenetic markers [24]. This is an important finding when one considers previous positive reports that were generated in retrospective, small series [25, 26]. An association between therapeutic outcome and variations in the CARD 15 (NOD2) gene can also be rejected with the necessary statistical power on the basis of the two-cohort design described above [27]. This is in agreement with a study of an outpatient population where no association could be found between NOD2 variations and outcome [28] but a decision between "a true negative finding" and "lack of power" is not allowed by the study design. The variations in the NOD2 gene, which were tested (G908R; R702W, '3020insC) are considered primary etiologic factors for the development of Crohn's disease [29-31].

Side effects

Immunosuppression leading to clinical benefits is accompanied by sometimes severe side-effects, which apparently relate to the very effect of the drug [32]. These side-effects include the occurrence of infectious complications including sepsis and tuberculosis [33, 34]. Therefore, the use of immunosuppressive agents should be preceded by adequate screening procedures and – if necessary – the appropriate anti-infective treatment or prophylaxis. An enhanced development of malignant diseases including lymphoma in patients who received treatment with infliximab has been suggested. This has not been evident in larger case series as observed malignancy rates do not statistically differ from those expected in the general population [35].

Immunization against foreign protein is a problem inherent to the application of recombinant proteins. The extent of murine sequence may be one predictor for immunogenicity. However, as even completely "human" proteins include neo-determinants (that are not previously known to the immune systems), it is somewhat difficult to predict immunogenicity for new compounds. The main problem is not that of adverse drug reaction at the time of infusion (acute infusion reactions) or in the days thereafter (delayed hypersensitivity, type IV "serum sickness" reaction) as this can be managed in most cases by standard care interventions including glucocorticoids, H1 antagonists and alpha-adrenergic substances. However, patients who frequently receive recombinant proteins as a last resort are most likely rendered unresponsive to future treatments with that particular drug if they have been immunized.

Future developments

Partitioning of Crohn's disease

With the discovery of the first disease gene in Crohn's disease (NOD2) [29-31], it has become clear that Crohn's disease itself is a syndrome rather than a single condition, in which several genes in combination determine complex phenotypes and – perhaps – response to some drugs. It is expected that additional disease genes are located on chromosome 16 in the "IBD1" susceptibility area [36], chromosome 6 ("IBD3") [7, 37-41], chromosome 12 ("IBD2") [39, 40-42], chromosome 4 ("IBD4") [39, 43] and chromosome 5 [44] among others. The next steps in molecular exploration will broaden our understanding of the interplay between different genetic susceptibility factors in this disease, and may identify genetic variations, which may exclusively determine response to specific anti-inflammatory treatments.

Other targets

Crohn's disease has become a playing field for pharmaceutical developments, which subsequently aim at larger markets such as rheumatoid arthritis and psoriasis. A host of potential drug targets has become available, with animal models having a limited capacity to identify the most promising ones. The tempting advantage of having an efficacy parameter as clear as mucosal inflammation has led to the introduction of appropriate and less appropriate experimental biological therapies at early stages of drug development in patients. However, one should be aware when assessing the risk-benefit-ratio that Crohn's disease leads to a sharp reduction in the quality of life during active phases, but does not result in a general decrease in life-expectancy in usually young patients.

The past few years have seen the discovery of many immune relevant drug targets which include immunologic mediators (*e.g.* IL-1, IL-6, IL-8, IL-12, IL-16, IL-18), transcription factors (*e.g.* NFkB, OCT-1, STAT-1, T-bet), adhesion molecules (*e.g.* ICAM-1, alpha 4-beta 7 integrin), cell cycle regulating factors (*e.g.* CD40/CD40-L, OX-40, OX-40L), proliferation associated enzymes (*e.g.* various kinases) amongst many others. In most cases biologicals have been developed to inhibit or modulate these target genes and proteins.

A particularly interesting case is interleukin-10 (IL-10). Interleukin-10 (IL-10), which was identified in 1989 as "cytokine synthesis inhibitory factor", profoundly inhibits effector functions of activated macrophages and monocytes *in vitro (Figure 2)* [45]. Interleukin-10 down-regulates the production of pro-inflammatory cytokines, interferon-γ and, to a lesser extent, IL-2 production by type 1 T-helper cells [46]. In various *in vitro* and *in vivo* models, interleukin-10 shows a strong anti-inflammatory effect [47-49]. This effect may be mediated by inhibition of the activation of nuclear factor kappa B [50-52], a transcription factor, which initiates or augments the expression of many pro-inflammatory mediators. Glucocorticoids exert some of their anti-inflammatory actions in a similar manner as interleukin-10, by inhibition of the activation of nuclear factor kappa B [53, 54].

Interleukin-10 is involved in the maintenance of the normal non-inflammatory state of the intestine [55]. Interleukin-10 also inhibits *in vitro* the pro-inflammatory activities of mononuclear cells which have been isolated from the intestinal *lamina propria* of patients with inflammatory bowel disease [48]. Clinical studies have suggested that interleukin-10 has some therapeutic activity in mild to moderate, untreated Crohn's disease [56]. However, in a large trial in chronic active, steroid-refractory Crohn's disease only limited clinical effects were seen [57] and promising data from an earlier pilot study in this condition could not be confirmed [58]. In a blinded subanalysis of the 329 patients included into the trial, it appeared that a responder subpopulation with a distinct downregulation of the NFkB system was present [57]. Unfortunately, a pharmacogenetic substudy was not part of the development program.

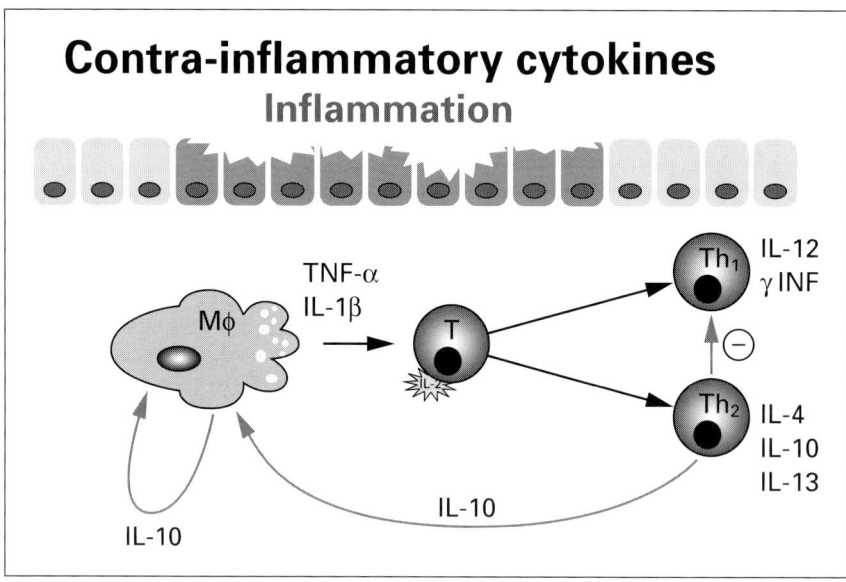

Figure 2. Anti-inflammatory action of human recombinant interleukin-10.

The clinical response to IL-10 followed a bell shaped dose-response curve with higher doses of IL-10 leading to a reduced clinical efficacy. This appeared mainly due to side effects including anemia (which is part of the CDAI), through the induction of gamma-interferon and other immunoregulatory cytokines [59]. While a systemic application of high doses of IL-10 may be not suitable, the topical application [48] is currently revisited. Possible genetic approaches, which have generated promising preclinical data, include the use of IL-10 producing lactobacilli [60] or of gut-homing T cells, that are isolated from peripheral blood and transfected with an IL-10 construct *ex vivo* before they are re-infused [61]. Both approaches will generate high mucosal levels of IL-10 and the first clinical results are expected with great interest.

The most promising new drug developments which approach the approval process are monoclonal antibodies which are directed against the integrin system (*e.g.* natalizumab directed against alpha4-integrin) and beta-interferon. It also appears important to reassess recombinant interleukin-1 receptor antagonist (IL-1ra, anakinra) as this molecule apparently failed a small trial for Crohn's disease (results were not published) but has shown strong signs of clinical efficacy in rheumatoid arthritis [62]. Many other novel agents which have either failed or are in the early stages of clinical development have been recently reviewed in detail [63].

The next generation of therapies

While a host of therapeutic trials has been launched or is currently being prepared using recombinant proteins to antagonise targets, the first new targeted developments return to orally available small molecules. A particular interesting concept is the introduction of orally available antisense-oligonucleotides which could block the mucosal production of TNF (*orasense* by ISIS Pharmaceuticals). However, this compound is still in the early stages of clinical research. Other developments include the refinement of anti-TNF compounds that are based on thalidomide. Thalidomide, approved in many markets for the therapy of lepra [64], has shown some signs of a clinical effect in small trials in Crohn's disease [65, 66]. Several orally avalaible TNF receptor antagonists are in the last stage of preclinical development.

A good example for a targeted development of an oral compound using combinatorial chemistry is the inhibition of MAP-kinase p38, as this molecule has revealed to be a relevant proximal regulator of TNF expression in Crohn's disease and other autoimmune conditions. Here, a designer drug approach has been adopted to generate a series of small molecule specific inhibitors [67], which are currently making their way into clinical phase II trials in Crohn's disease, rheumatoid arthritis and psoriasis.

Outlook

Crohn's disease therapy is a field that will witness the successful development of biological drugs that probably result in potent beneficial effects in patient subpopulations. Biological drugs will map targets that will be addressed by subsequent developments of orally available small-molecule compounds. The progress in IBD therapy outlines how the findings that have come about from the present genomic revolution can be used. However the real test to the value of genomic insights that are generated in IBD will be the effect of novel drug on the long-term quality of life of the patients.

The induction of mucosal healing by infliximab, which cannot be achieved with glucocorticoids, or requires a long time treatment with azathioprine (if successful at all), results in a slow but steady redefinition of remission as a clinical endpoint in the general approach to the disease. It is therefore anticipated that future clinical developments will have to address remission rather than response as a clinical endpoint. The definition of remission may have to include endoscopic healing (which is not well defined as of yet [68]) in addition to clinical improvement (CDAI<150) as mucosal recovery may be associated with a favorable mid-term prognosis [69].

It is the sincere hope that these developments are accompanied by the definition of molecular markers that help to predict the selective response to some of the drugs. The future of Crohn's disease therapy cannot evolve to a try-and-error scheme using various recombinant, parenteral therapies but rather has to develop into a rational use compounds including oral drugs.

Acknowledgements

The work described in this chapter was partially supported by grants from the BMBF (Competence Network Inflammatory Bowel Disease, German National Genome Research

Network) and the Deutsche Forschungsgemeinschaft. Parts of the text have appeared in similar form in the *Annals of Gastroenterology*.

References

1. MacDonald TT, Hutchings P, Choy MY, Murch S, Cooke A. Tumour necrosis factor-alpha and interferon-gamma production measured at the single cell level in normal and inflamed human intestine. *Clin Exp Immunol* 1990; 81: 301-5.
2. Reinecker HC, Steffen M, Witthoeft T, Pflueger I, Schreiber S, MacDermott RP, Raedler A. Enhanced secretion of tumour necrosis factor-alpha, IL-6, and IL-1 beta by isolated lamina propria mononuclear cells from patients with ulcerative colitis and Crohn's disease. *Clin Exp Immunol* 1993; 94: 174-81.
3. Schreiber S, Nikolaus S, Hampe J, Hämling J, Koop I, Groessner B, Lochs H, Raedler A. Tumor necrosis factor-a and interleukin-1ß in relapse of Crohn's disease. *Lancet* 1999, 353: 459-61.
4. Hampe J, Shaw SH, Saiz R, Leysens N, Lantermann A, Mascheretti S, Lynch NJ, MacPherson AJ, Bridger S, van Deventer S, Stokkers P, Morin P, Mirza MM, Forbes A, Lennard-Jones JE, Mathew CG, Curran ME, Schreiber S. Linkage of inflammatory bowel disease to human chromosome 6p. *Am J Hum Genet* 1999; 65: 1647-55.
5. Bouma G, Crusius JB, Oudkerk-Pool M, Kolkman JJ, von Blomberg BM, Kostense PJ, *et al.* Secretion of tumour necrosis factor alpha and lymphotoxin alpha in relation to polymorphisms in the TNF genes and HLA-DR alleles. Relevance for inflammatory bowel disease. *Scand J Immunol* 1996; 43: 456-63.
6. Beutler B. Autoimmunity and apoptosis: the Crohn's connection. *Immunity* 2001; 15: 5-14.
7. van Dullemen HM, van Deventer SJH, Hommes DW, Bijl HA, Jansen J, Tytgat GNJ, Woody J. Treatment of Crohn's disease with anti-tumor necrosis factor chimeric antibody (cA2). *Gastroenterology* 1995; 109: 129-35.
8. Targan SR, Hanauer SB, van Deventer SJH, Mayer L, Present DH, Braakman T, de Woody KL, Schaible TF, Rutgeerts PJ. A short-term study of chimeric monoclonal antibody cA2 to tumor necrosis factorα for Crohn's disease. *N Engl J Med* 1997; 337: 1029-35.
9. Nikolaus S, Raedler A, Sfikas N, Kühbacher T, Fölsch UR, Schreiber S. Mechanisms in failure of infliximab for Crohn's disease. *Lancet* 2000; 356: 1475-9.
10. Schreiber S, Campieri M, Colombel JF, van Deventer SJH, Feagan B, Fedorak R, Forbes A, Gassull M, Gendre JP, van Hogezand RA, Lofberg R, Modigliani R, Pallone F, Petritsch W, Prantera C, Rampton D, Seibold F, Vatn M, Zeitz M, Rutgeerts P. Use of anti-tumour necrosis factor agents in inflammatory bowel disease. European guidelines for 2001-2003. *Int J Colorectal Dis* 2001; 16: 1-11.
11. Hanauer SB, Feagan BG, Lichtenstein GR, Mayer LF, Schreiber S, Colombel JF, Rachmilewitz D, Wolf DC, Olson A, Bao W, Rutgeerts P. Maintenance infliximab for Crohn's disease: the ACCENT I randomized trial. *Lancet* 2002; 359: 1541-9.
12. Sands WJ, van Deventer S, Bernstein C, Kamm M, Rachmilewitz D, Chey W, Lashner B, Wolf D, Blank M, Wild G, Fedorak R, Feagan B, Anderson F, Marster P, Rutgeerts P. Long-term treatment of fistulizing Crohn's disease: response to infliximab in the ACCENT II trial through 54 weeks. *Gastroenterology* 2002; 122: A81 (abstract).
13. Probert CSJ, Hearing SD, Schreiber S, Kühbacher T, Ghosh S, Arnott IDR, Forbes A. Infliximab in glucocorticoid-resistant ulcerative colitis – a randomized controlled trial. Submitted.
14. Sandborn WJ, Hanauer SB, Katz S, Safdi M, Wolf DG, Baerg RD, Tremaine WJ, Johnson T, Diehl NN, Zinsmeister AR. Etanercept for active Crohn's disease: a randomized, double-blind, placebo-controlled trial. *Gastroenterology* 2001; 121: 1088-94.

15. Stack WA, Mann SD, Roy AJ, Heath P, Sopwith M, Freeman J, Holmes G, Long R, Forbes A, Kamm MA. Randomised controlled trial of CDP571 antibody to tumour necrosis factor-alpha in Crohn's disease. *Lancet* 1997; 22: 521-4.
16. Kriegler M, Perez C, DeFay K, Albert I, Lu SD. A novel form of TNF/cachectin is a cell surface cytotoxic transmembrane protein: ramifications for the complex physiology of TNF. *Cell* 1988; 53: 45-53.
17. Waetzig G, Seegert D, Rosenstiel P, Nikolaus N, Schreiber S. p38 mitogen-activated protein kinase is activated and linked to TNF-alpha signaling in inflammatory bowel disease. *J Immunol* 2002; 168: 5342-51.
18. Scallon BJ, Moore MA, Trinh DM, Ghrayeb J. Chimeric anti-TNF-a monoclonal antibody, cA2, binds recombinant transmembrane TNF-a and activates immune effector functions. *Cytokine* 1995; 7: 251-9.
19. ten Hove T, van Montfrans C, Peppelenbosch MP, van Deventer SJ. Infliximab treatment induces apoptosis of lamina propria T lymphocytes in Crohn's disease. *Gut* 2002; 50: 206-11.
20. Lugering A, Schmidt M, Lugering N, Pauels HG, Domschke W, Kucharzik T. Infliximab induces apoptosis in monocytes from patients with chronic active Crohn's disease by using a caspase-dependent pathway. *Gastroenterology* 2001; 121: 1145-57.
21. Mascheretti S, Hampe J, Kühbacher T, Herfarth H, Krawczak M, Fölsch UR, Schreiber S. Pharmacogenetic investigation of the TNF/TNF-receptor system in patients with chronic active Crohn's disease treated with infliximab. *Pharmacogenomics J* 2002; 2: 127-36.
22. Taylor KD, Plevy SE, Yang H, Landers CJ, Barry MJ, Rotter JI, et al. ANCA pattern and LTA haplotype relationships to clinical responses to anti-TNF antibody treatment in Crohn's disease. *Gastroenterology* 2001; 120: 1347-55.
23. Vermeire S, Monsuur F, Groenen P, Peeters M, Vlietinck R, Rutgeerts P. Response to anti-TNFa treatment is associated with the TNFa-308*1 allele. *Gastroenterology* 2000; 118: A654.
24. Mascheretti S, Hampe J, Croucher PJP, Nikolaus S, Andus T, Schubert S, Olson A, Bao W, Fölsch UR, Schreiber S. Response to infliximab treatment in Crohn's disease is not associated with mutations in the CARD15 (NOD2) gene. *J Pharmacogenetics* 2002, in press.
25. Vermeire S, Louis E, Rutgeerts P, De Vos M, Van Gossum A, Belaiche J, Pescatore P, Fiasse R, Pelckmans P, Vlietinck R, Merlin F, Zouali H, Thomas G, Colombel JF, Hugot JP. Belgian Group of Infliximab Expanded Access Program and Fondation Jean Dausset CEPH, Paris, France. NOD2/CARD15 does not influence response to infliximab in Crohn's disease. *Gastroenterology* 2002; 123: 106-11.
26. Hugot JP, Chamaillard M, Zouali H, Lesage S, Cezard JP, Belaiche J, Almer S, Tysk C, O'Morain CA, Gassull M, Binder V, Finkel Y, Cortot A, Modigliani R, Laurent-Puig P, Gower-Rousseau C, Macry J, Colombel JF, Sahbatou M, Thomas G. Association of NOD2 leucine-rich repeat variants with susceptibility to Crohn's disease. *Nature* 2001; 411: 599-603.
27. Ogura Y, Bonen DK, Inohara N, Nicolae DL, Chen FF, Ramos R, Britton H, Moran T, Karaliuskas R, Duerr RH, Achkar JP, Brant SR, Bayless TM, Kirschner BS, Hanauer SB, Nunez G, Cho JH. A frameshift mutation in NOD2 associated with susceptibility to Crohn's disease. *Nature* 2001; 411: 603-6.
28. Hampe J, Cuthbert A, Croucher PJ, Mirza MM, Mascheretti S, Fisher S, Frenzel H, King K, Hasselmeyer A, MacPherson AJ, Bridger S, van Deventer S, Forbes A, Nikolaus S, Lennard-Jones JE, Foelsch UR, Krawczak M, Lewis C, Schreiber S, Mathew CG. Association between insertion mutation in NOD2 gene and Crohn's disease in German and British populations. *Lancet* 2001; 357: 1925-8.
29. Aithal GP, Mansfield JC. Review article: the risk of lymphoma associated with inflammatory bowel disease and immunosuppressive treatment. *Aliment Pharmacol Ther* 2001; 15: 1101-8.

30. Nunez Martinez O, Ripoll Noiseux C, Carneros Martin JA, Gonzalez Lara V, Gregorio Maranon HG. Reactivation tuberculosis in a patient with anti-TNF-alpha treatment. *Am J Gastroenterol* 2001; 96: 1665-6.
31. Keane J, Gershon S, Wise RP, Mirabile-Levens E, Kasznica J, Schwieterman WD, Siegel JN, Braun MM. Tuberculosis associated with infliximab, a tumor necrosis factor alpha-neutralizing agent. *N Engl J Med* 2001; 345: 1098-104.
32. Bickston SJ, Lichtenstein GR, Arseneau KO, Cohen RB, Cominelli F. The relationship between infliximab treatment and lymphoma in Crohn's disease. *Gastroenterology* 1999; 117: 1433-7.
33. Hampe J, Frenzel H, Mirza MM, Croucher PJP, Cuthbert A, Mascheretti S, Huse K, Platzer M, Bridger S, Meyer B, Nürnberg P, Stokkers P, Krawczak M, Mathew CG, Curran M, Schreiber S. Evidence for a NOD2 independent susceptibility locus for inflammatory bowel disease on chromosome 16p. *Proc Natl Acad Sci USA* 2002; 99: 321-6.
34. Rioux JD, Silverberg MS, Daly MJ, *et al.* Genomewide search in Canadian families with inflammatory bowel disease reveals two novel susceptibility loci. *Am J Hum Genet* 2000; 66: 1863-70.
35. Satsangi J, Welsh KI, Bunce M, Julier C, Farrant JM, Bell JI, Jewell DP. Contribution of genes of the major histocompatibility complex to susceptibility and disease phenotype in inflammatory bowel disease. *Lancet* 1996; 347: 1212-7.
36. Hampe J, Schreiber S, Shaw S, Lau KF, Bridger S, Macpherson AJS, Cardon LR, Sakul H, Harris TJR, Buckler A, Hall J, Stokkers P, van Deventer SJH, Nurnberg P, Mirza M, Lee J, Lennard-Jones JE, Mathew C, Curran ME. A genomewide analysis provides evidence for novel linkages in inflammatory bowel disease in a large European cohort. *Am J Hum Genet* 1999; 64: 808-16.
37. Satsangi J, Parkes M, Louis E, Hashimoto L, Kato N, Welsh K, Terwilliger JD, *et al.* Two stage genome-wide search in inflammatory bowel disease provides evidence for susceptibility loci on chromosomes 3, 7 and 12. *Nat Genet* 1996; 14: 199-202.
38. Duerr RH, Barnada M, Zhang L, *et al.* Linkage and association between inflammatory bowel disease and a locus on chromosome 12. *Am J Hum Genet* 1998; 63: 95-100.
39. Yang H, Ohmen JD, Ma Y, Bentley LG, Targan SR, Fischel-Ghodsian N, Rotter JI. Additional evidence of linkage between Crohn's disease and a putative locus on chromosome 12. *Genet Med* 1999; 1: 194-8.
40. Cho JH, Nicolae DL, Gold LH, Fields CT, LaBuda MC, Rohal PM, Pickles MR, Qin L, Fu Y, Mann JS, Kirschner BS, Jabs EW, Weber J, Hanauer SB, Bayless TM, Brant SR. Identification of novel susceptibility loci for inflammatory bowel disease on chromosomes 1p, 3q, and 4q: evidence for epistasis between 1p and IBD1. *Proc Natl Acad Sci USA* 1998; 95: 7502-7.
41. Rioux JD, Daly MJ, Silverberg MS, Lindblad K, Steinhart H, Cohen Z, Delmonte T, Kocher K, Miller K, Guschwan S, Kulbokas EJ, O'Leary S, Winchester E, Dewar K, Green T, Stone V, Chow C, Cohen A, Langelier D, Lapointe G, Gaudet D, Faith J, Branco N, Bull SB, McLeod RS, Griffiths AM, Bitton A, Greenberg GR, Lander ES, Siminovitch KA, Hudson TJ. Genetic variation in the 5q31 cytokine gene cluster confers susceptibility to Crohn disease. *Nat Genet* 2001; 29: 223-8.
42. de Waal Malefyt R, Yssel H, Roncarolo MG, Spits H, de Vries JE. Interleukin-10. *Curr Opin Immunol* 1992; 4: 314-22.
43. Fiorentino DF, Bond MW, Mosmann TR. Two types of mouse T helper cells. IV. Th2 clones secrete a factor that inhibits cytokine production by Th1 clones. *J Exp Med* 1989; 170: 2081-95.
44. Pajkrt D, Camoglio L, Tiel-van Buul MC, de Bruin K, Cutler DL, Affrime MB, Rikken G, van der Poll T, ten Cate JW, van Deventer SJ. Attenuation of proinflammatory response by recombinant human IL-10 in human endotoxemia: effect of timing of recombinant human IL-10 administration. *J Immunol* 1997; 158: 3971-7.
45. Schreiber S, Heinig T, Thiele HG, Raedler A. Immunoregulatory role of interleukin-10 in patients with inflammatory bowel disease. *Gastroenterology* 1995; 108: 1434-44.

46. Asadullah K, Sterry W, Stephanek K, Jasulaitis D, Leupold M, Audring H, Volk HD, Docke WD. IL-10 is a key cytokine in psoriasis. Proof of principle by IL-10 therapy: a new therapeutic approach. *J Clin Invest* 1998; 101: 783-94.
47. Wang P, Wu P, Siegel MI, Egan RW, Billah MM. Interleukin (IL)-10 inhibits nuclear factor kappa B (NF kappa B) activation in human monocytes. IL-10 and IL-4 suppress cytokine synthesis by different mechanisms. *J Biol Chem* 1995; 270: 9558-63.
48. Schreiber S, Nikolaus S, Hampe J. Activation of nuclear factor kappa B in inflammatory bowel disease. *Gut* 1998; 42: 477-85.
49. Schottelius AJ, Mayo MW, Sartor RB, Baldwin AS Jr. Interleukin-10 signaling blocks inhibitor of kappa B kinase activity and nuclear factor kappa B DNA binding. *J Biol Chem* 1999; 274: 31868-74.
50. Scheinman RI, Cogswell PC, Lofquist AK, Baldwin AS Jr. Role of transcriptional activation by IkB in mediation of immunosuppression by glucocorticoids. *Science* 1995; 270: 283-6.
51. Auphan N, DiDonato JA, Rosette C, Helmberg A, Karin M. Immunosuppression by glucocorticoids: inhibition of NFkB activity through induction of IkB synthesis. *Science* 1995; 270: 286-90.
52. Kühn R, Löhler J, Rennick D, Rajewsky K, Müller W. Interleukin-10-deficient mice develop chronic enterocolitis. *Cell* 1993; 75: 263-74.
53. Fedorak RN, Gangl A, Elson CO, Rutgeerts P, Schreiber S, Wild G, Hanauer SB, Kilian A, Cohard M, LeBeaut A, Feagan B. Recombinant human interleukin-10 in the treatment of patients with mild to moderately active Crohn's disease. *Gastroenterology* 2000; 119: 1473-82.
54. Schreiber S, Fedorak RN, Nielsen OH, Wild G, Williams NC, Nikolaus S, Jacyna M, Lashner BA, Gangl A, Rutgeerts P, Isaacs K, van Deventer SJH, Koningsberger JC, Cohard M, Lebeaut A, Hanauer SB. Recombinant human interleukin-10 in active Crohn's disease. *Gastroenterology* 2000; 119: 1461-72.
55. Van Deventer SJ, Elson CO, Fedorak RN. Multiple doses of intravenous interleukin-10 in patients with inflammatory bowel disease. *Gastroenterology* 1997; 1113: 383-9.
56. Tilg H, van Montfrans C, van Den Ende A, Kaser A, van Deventer SJ, Schreiber S, Gregor M, Ludwiczek O, Rutgeerts P, Gasche C, Koningsberger JC, Abreu L, Kuhn I, Cohard M, LeBeaut A, Grint P, Weiss G. Treatment of Crohn's disease with recombinant human interleukin-10 induces the proinflammatory cytokine interferon gamma. *Gut* 2002; 50: 191-5.
57. Steidler L, Hans W, Schotte L, Neirynck S, Obermeier F, Falk W, Fiers W, Remaut E. Treatment of murine colitis by *Lactococcus lactis* secreting interleukin-10. *Science* 2000; 289: 1352-5.
58. Van Deventer SJ. The future of inflammatory bowel disease therapy. *Inflamm Bowel Dis* 2002; 8: 301-5.
59. Jiang Y, Genant HK, Watt I, Cobby M, Bresnihan B, Aitchison R, McCabe D. A multicenter, double-blind, dose-ranging, randomized, placebo-controlled study of recombinant human interleukin-1 receptor antagonist in patients with rheumatoid arthritis: radiologic progression and correlation of Genant and Larsen scores. *Arthritis Rheum* 2000; 43: 1001-9.
60. Sandborn WJ, Targan SR. Biologic therapy of inflammatory bowel disease. *Gastroenterology* 2002; 122: 1592-608.
61. Iyer CG, Languillon J, Ramanujam K, Tarabini-Castellani G, De las Aguas JT, Bechelli LM, Uemura K, Martinez Dominguez V, Sundaresan T. WHO co-ordinated short-term double-blind trial with thalidomide in the treatment of acute lepra reactions in male lepromatous patients. *Bull WHO* 1971; 45: 719-32.
62. Vasiliauskas EA, Kam LY, Abreu-Martin MT, Hassard PV, Papadakis KA, Yang H, Zeldis JB, Targan SR. An open-label pilot study of low-dose thalidomide in chronically active, steroid-dependent Crohn's disease. *Gastroenterology* 1999; 117: 1278-87.
63. Ehrenpreis ED, Kane SV, Cohen LB, Cohen RD, Hanauer SB. Thalidomide therapy for patients with refractory Crohn's disease: an open-label trial. *Gastroenterology* 1999; 117: 1271-7.

64. Pargellis C, Tong L, Churchill L, Cirillo PF, Gilmore T, Graham AG, Grob PM, Hickey ER, Moss N, Pav S, Regan J. Inhibition of p38 MAP kinase by utilizing a novel allosteric binding site. *Nat Struct Biol* 2002; 9: 268-72.
65. Cellier C, Sahmoud T, Froguel E, Adenis A, Belaiche J, Bretagne JF, Florent C, Bouvry M, Mary JY, Modigliani R. Correlations between clinical activity, endoscopic severity, and biological parameters in colonic or ileocolonic Crohn's disease. A prospective multicentre study of 121 cases. The Groupe d'Études Thérapeutiques des Affections Inflammatoires Digestives. *Gut* 1994; 35: 231-5.
66. Allez M, Lemann M, Bonnet J, Cattan P, Jian R, Modigliani R. Long-term outcome of patients with active Crohn's disease exhibiting extensive and deep ulcerations at colonoscopy. *Am J Gastroenterol* 2002; 97: 947-53.
67. Pargellis C, Tong L, Churchill L, Cirillo PF, Gilmore T, Graham AG, Grob PM, Hickey ER, Moss N, Pav S, Regan J. Inhibition of p38 MAP kinase by utilizing a novel allosteric binding site. *Nat Struct Biol* 2002; 9: 268-72.
68. Cellier C, Sahmoud T, Froguel E, Adenis A, Belaiche J, Bretagne JF, Florent C, Bouvry M, Mary JY, Modigliani R. Correlations between clinical activity, endoscopic severity, and biological parameters in colonic or ileocolonic Crohn's disease. A prospective multicentre study of 121 cases. The Groupe d'Études Thérapeutiques des Affections Inflammatoires Digestives. *Gut* 1994; 35: 231-5.
69. Allez M, Lemann M, Bonnet J, Cattan P, Jian R, Modigliani R. Long-term outcome of patients with active Crohn's disease exhibiting extensive and deep ulcerations at colonoscopy. *Am J Gastroenterol* 2002; 97: 974-53.

Irritable bowel syndrome and other functional bowel disorders. New answers to old questions

Paul Enck, Heinemarie Hinninghofen

Department of General Surgery, University Hospitals Tübingen, Germany

Visceral hyperalgesia: a new pathophysiological understanding of functional bowel disorders

Thirty years ago, hypersensitivity of the bowel towards experimental balloon distension has for the first time been demonstrated experimentally in patients with the irritable bowel syndrome (IBS) [1] as compared to healthy controls and was assumed to be a major clinical feature in these diseases. However, other mechanisms such as hyper- or hypomotility of the colon or other compartments of the gastrointestinal tract [2, 3], psychoneurotism [4], excessive stress responsivenesss [5], and other pathophysiological hypotheses have been tested during subsequent years, and have been approved or disapproved as relevant for symptom occurrence and severity in functional bowel disorders, especially in IBS (for a review of these early day studies, see [6]). Similar discussions – and experimental testings – were also held for upper gastrointestinal complaints of functional origin, for what is today labelled "functional dyspepsia" (FD) and "non-cardiac-chest pain" (NCCP).

It was the international effort to standardize not only nomenclature and clinical definitions, but also the way functional gastrointestinal disorders are diagnosed and managed clinically – known as the Rome criteria – which marked the beginning of a new understanding of functional bowel disorders. The Rome criteria – first published in 1988 [7] based in the preceding Manning criteria [8] – not only summarized the collected evidence for underlying pathomechanisms of these functional disorders, but also generated a series of new experiments especially with respect to the pathogenesis of IBS, FD, and NCCP. As one of the consequences, it is agreed by most clinicians and experts today that hypersensitivity of gut compartments towards physiological stimuli which are perceived as painful is the only pathomechanism which carries significant scientific evidence [9-14]. *Figure 1* illustrates the major findings of two such studies with similar approaches. Subsequent Rome (II) criteria revisions and extensions [15] have not changed this basic concept.

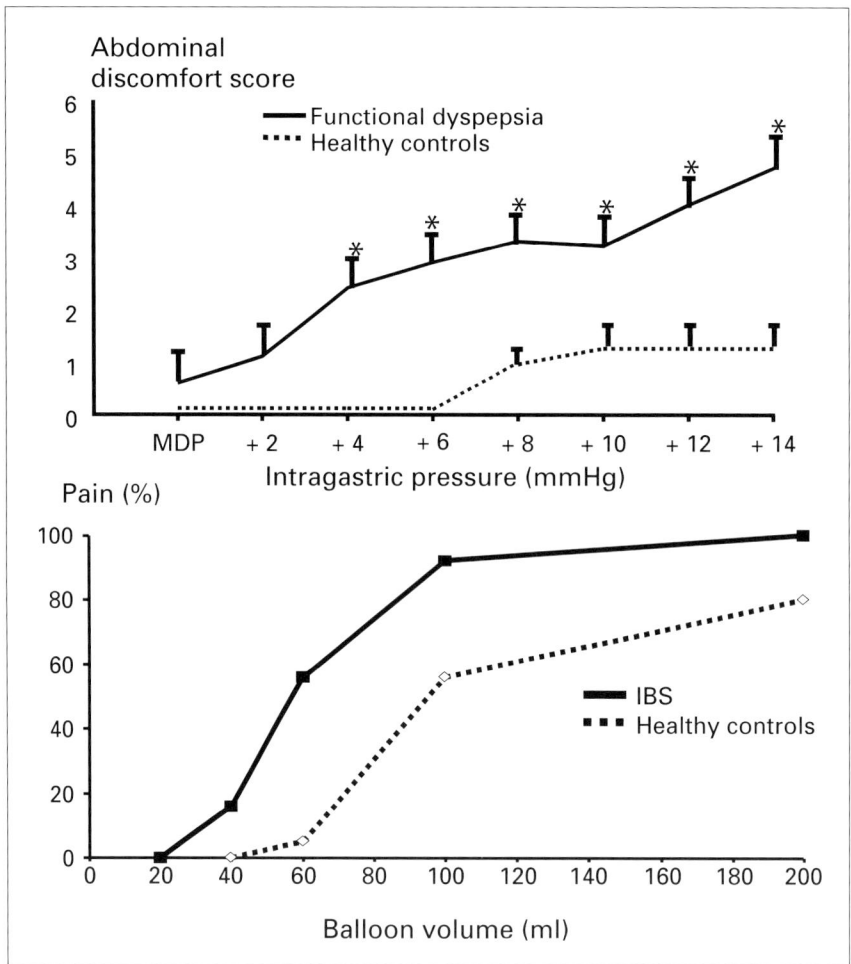

Figure 1. Visceral hypersensitivity towards experimental balloon distension of the esophagus, stomach, and colon in two studies [9, 14] – in each case, the cumulative response curve (% pain responses) of patients with functional bowel disorders (FD, IBS) is shifted to the left as compared to healthy volunteers indicating hypersentivitiy to stimuli non-painful in normal conditions.

The open question No. 1: Where is visceral hyperalgesia located?

Proof that a patient with IBS has "visceral hyperalgesia" – *i.e.* that he/she reports intestinal events as painful which others may not recognize at all – may be sufficient for the patient to understand his/her symptoms, and may even allow a physician to improve clinical management of the patient, but it leaves one central question unanswered: where is the hyperalgesia located? Is it a local event at the level of the gut wall or lumen, or a central event at the spinal or cortical level? In the last decade, evidence has been gathered for all three possibilities – a final conclusion has not yet been reached.

Local

Gross macroscopic abnormalities of the gut wall are excluded by definition in functional bowel disorders; this also excludes inflammatory processes at a microscopic level. Alterations of bowel wall elasticity (compliance), as it can be found in patients with inflammatory bowel disorders (colitis, Crohn's disease) even in asymptomatic periods of the disease [16], have also been excluded in functional bowel disorders.

However, recent findings indicate that mucosal biopsies in IBS patients contain increased levels of mast cells [17-19], neuropeptides [20], and enterochromafin cells [21] as compared to healthy subjects, but lower levels as they are usually found in patients with acute inflammation *(Figure 2)*. In other studies, mucosal cytokines were downregulated in IBS as compared to controls [22]. This indicates that at the gut lumen or wall level biochemical indicators exist which points towards a history of inflammation in these patients. A previous inflammation is reported frequently by many patients during anamnesis.

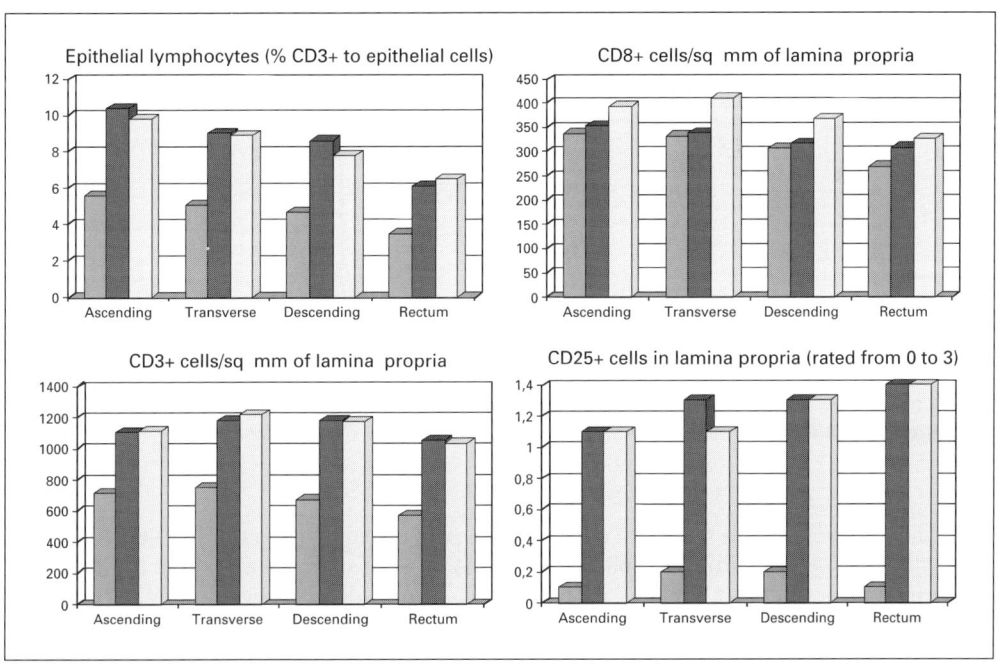

Figure 2. Increased release of neuroendocrine cells in patients with post-desynteric IBS-like symptoms as compared to patients with acute inflammation and to normal healthy controls (data from: 19).

Spinal

Repetitive stimulation, *e.g.* balloon distension of one gut segment, leads to increased sensitivity towards distension of the respective segment, but also adjacent segments not directly affected by the procedure [23]. Acid exposure of the lower esophagus increases the sensitivity of the upper esophagus also for electrical stimulation [24], and changes cortical processing of visceral sensations [25]. Experimentally increased sensitivity of the gut is also reflected by an increased abdominal referral area both in animals [26] and in men [27].

Increased abdominal referral area following intestinal stimulation was already noted by Ritchie in 1973 [1] as one of the major features of IBS patients, and this finding has been replicated recently [23]. It is also known for other functional bowel disorders and other gastrointestinal compartments *(Figure 3)*.

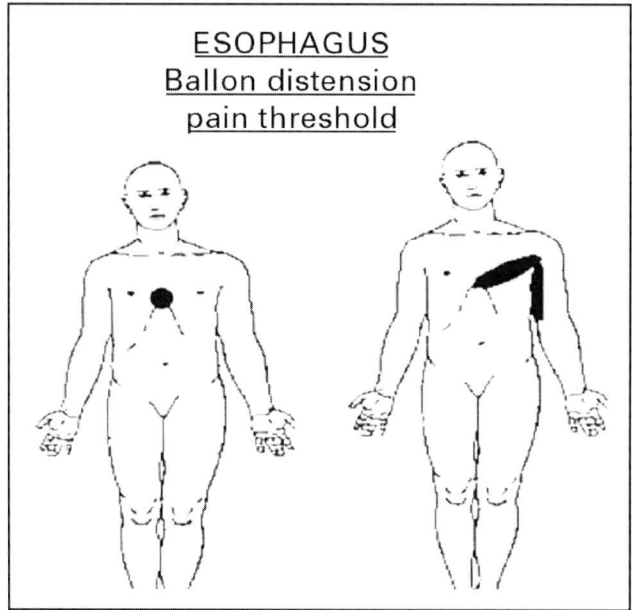

Figure 3. Increased referral area in a patient with functional non-cardiac chest pain as compared to a healthy subject following esophageal balloon distension with 10 ml of air.

This phenomenon is well known in experimental pain research as **secondary sensitization**: it is known to occur within the spinal cord at the level of dorsal horn where transmission of peripheral nociceptive input is modulated by central descending inhibitory pathways [28]. If a spinal "gate" has once been opened, it may eventually occur that a "pain memory" is formatted which will persist even after ceasing of the primary inflammatory process. Visceral hyperalgesia in functional bowel disorders is currently been thought to be generated that way.

Cortical

It has been well known for many years that patients with functional gastrointestinal disorders exhibit significant psychological and psychiatric disturbances [4]; however, increased scores on psychological tests are no primary markers of altered central processing of visceral sensations – they could also be secondary signs of clinical symptoms associated with visceral hyperalgesia.

The very first direct evidence for altered central processing of visceral sensations in IBS patients came from studies imaging brain activation during anticipated and true rectal stimulation [29]. It was shown in this and other studies [30-32] that in IBS patients activation of some areas of the brain such as the anterior cingulate gyrus are less pronounced (and less well correlated to stimulation intensity) than are other areas such as the prefrontal cortex.

These areas are not at all specific for visceral information processing but share this task with processing of nociceptive and aversive afferents from the body's periphery; however, the combination of specific areas activated following intestinal stimuli may well express a visceral, *e.g.* "anorectal brain network" [33] *(Figure 4)* whose spacial and timely organisation is not yet fully understood. A similar approach has been successful for the understanding of the central processing of micturition [34].

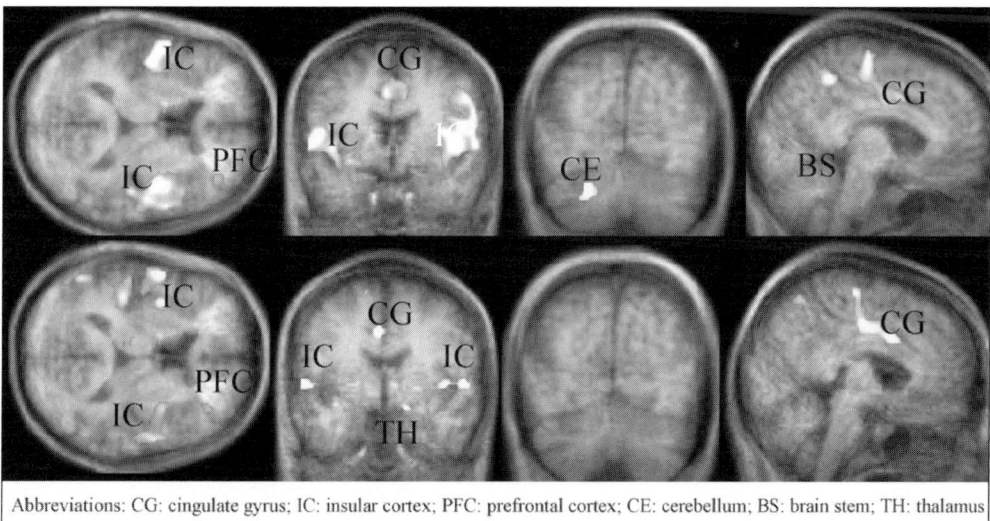

Abbreviations: CG: cingulate gyrus; IC: insular cortex; PFC: prefrontal cortex; CE: cerebellum; BS: brain stem; TH: thalamus

Figure 4. Anorectal "brain network" of areas activated with anal and rectal stimulation: activated areas include specific and unspecific components, both to painful and non-painful experimental stimuli of the lower GI tract (for details, see 33).

Open question No. 2:
How can visceral hyperalgesia occur?

Even if the properties of visceral hyperalgesia in patients with functional bowel disorders are about to be elucidated, as discussed above, and different clinical phenotypes are potentially relevant for different subtypes of patients within one clinical category (*e.g.* IBS), the exact pathophysiological mechanism how hyperalgesia in IBS is generated remains open to speculation, at least in individual patients. This is partly due to the fact that – as with many other diseases – the occurrence of IBS in any given healthy population can only be studied in large cohorts followed over a long period of time, depending on the overall prevalence of the disease, to generate a sufficient number of patients studies prospectively.

An alternative access was recently discovered with the occurrence of large-scale "epidemiological experiments" during endemic episodes of intestinal inflammation in communities, as reported below. They have further supported the notion that in a large group of patients with functional bowel disorders, a previous experience of a gastrointestinal inflammation of any kind may mark the beginning of the disease; this was reported anecdotally by many patients in the past, it even occasionally occurred in scientific papers (but left without final proof) [35], but was missing evidence until recently.

This has further supported the concept of a "central (spinal) sensitization" as the major underlying mechanisms in development of functional bowel disorders [4] *(see above)*. It has gained wide acceptance, but was lacking the final clinical proof in a prospective study; this gap was overcome with the studies reported here.

Quasi-experimental proof: post-infection IBS

The first prospective report of persistent of IBS-type symptoms after an acute episode of enteritis was reported by McKendrick anf Read [36] in 38 patients involved in two salmonella food poisoning events in a nursing home, and in 33 of these patients stool cultures had been shown to be positive for *Salmonella enteritidis* phage type 4. Clearance cultures were available from 28 patients, and all were negative. At time of food poisoning, none of the patients reported any history of chronic gastrointestinal complaints prior to it. Twelve months later, 12 of these patients had persistent bowel symptoms consistent with the diagnosis of IBS according to the Rome criteria, *i.e.* abdominal pain and altered stool habits without evidence for structural damage. All had been positive for salmonella, and 10 had had a negative clearance. Patients in whom IBS developed had had more severe symptoms during the acute disease.

A similar report by Gwee *et al.* [37] followed 75 patients with an episode of acute gastroenteritis admitted to a department of infectious diseases in Sheffield, England. Three months later, 22 reported persistent symptoms compatible with the diagnosis of IBS, and 3 more patients were symptomatic but did not match the diagnostic criteria. Twenty of the 22 were still symptomatic after 6 months, 15/19 at nine month and 9/12 after one year.

While symptom severity had been equal in those who did as to those who did not develop IBS, duration of diarrhea and abdominal pain during acute inflammation had been more pronounced in the IBS group.

The most recent report by Neal *et al.* [38] investigated 544 people with acute microbiologically confirmed bacterial gastroenteritis – due to campylobacter, salmonella or shigella – in Nottingham, England, by means of a symptom questionnaire six months after the event. They found 90/544 to be still symptomatic compared to before the illness, and 23 matched the Rome criteria after but not before the disease (new cases). Risk factors identified for them were sex and the duration of diarrhea during the acute episode.

The three reports yield a prevalence of post-infection IBS between 7 % and 30% of patients experiencing an acute bacterial infection at one point.

It remains to be shown whether other functional bowel disorders – FD and NCCP – resemble a similar pathomechanism at least for a substantial subgroup of patients: episodes of excessive esophageal acid reflux or symptomatic *Helicobacter* inflammation may be of similar importance in the disease history as is colonic inflammation in IBS [39].

Consequences for patient management in functional bowel disorders

One of the driving forces of this new development in our understanding of functional bowel disorders was the lack of appropriate medical treatment options for these diseases, especially the lack of drugs which target the gastrointestinal tract and its sensory and motor functions. New prokinetic compounds beyond cisapride were developed which addressed disturbed motility in different intestinal compartments, *e.g.* new 5-HT3 antagonists [40] and 5-HT4-agonists [41]. All have been shown to be effective in IBS, but it was speculated early that this effect was only partially due to the prokinetic action. A recent report demonstrated for the first time that *e.g.* tegaserod also exhibits anti-nociceptive effects on visceral afferents in animal models [42] which may become a major drug development target in the near future [43].

A second consequence of this new understanding of functional bowel disorders was the fact that – if abnormal central pain processing is a major issue – any therapeutic approach altering cortical processing of visceral afferent informations would be of clinical value, psychotherapy as much as "pain killers". It reestablished the relevance of different psychotherapy approaches which had shown in the past that they were superior to medical treatment alone, when combined with conventional medical management, irrespective of the specific psychological approach taken, *e.g.* hypnotherapy, behavioral management, cognitive therapy, or psychoanalysis [44].

All questions answered – and new ones generated

While post-infectious IBS has become a convincing example of how functional bowel disorders may occur after an acute episode of gastroenteritis, it cannot answer the puzzling fact that not all who experience enteritis once during their lifetime (and the lifetime prevalence is very high) do not develop post-infectious IBS, but only a minority of 20 % to 30%. In the above cited studies, neither the severity of the primary infectious disease *per se* nor other clinical data could predict the later-occurring IBS symptoms in a sugroup of patients.

However, in one of the studies [37] investigators had recorded psychometric test scores of patients immediately after the infectious disease outbreak, and long before it was evident which fraction of the patient would develop IBS symptoms months later. When these scores were compared between patients who developed IBS later and those who did not, significant differences arose with respect to anxiety, somatization, neuroticism, and hypochoindriasis *(Figure 5)*, and patients who became IBS sufferers 6 months later also had experienced more stressful life events at the time of assessment than their respective counterparts.

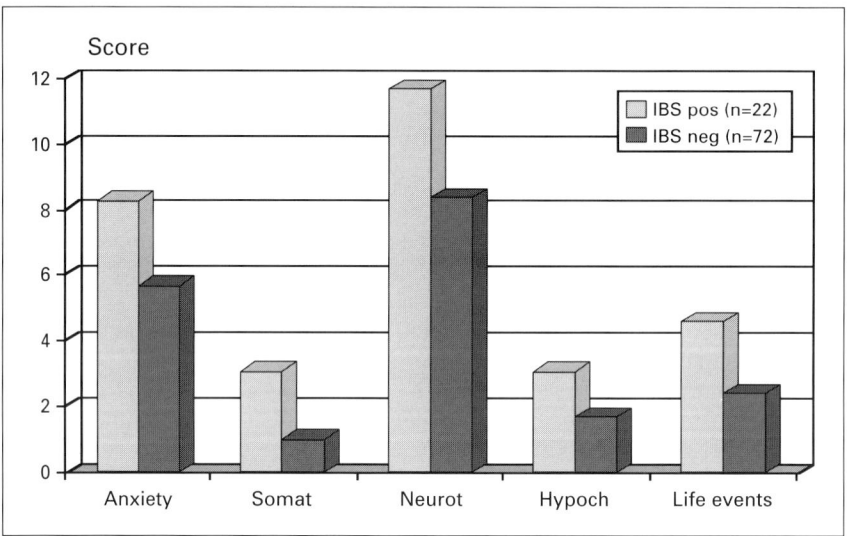

Figure 5. Psychological determinants of who would develop IBS symptoms following an acute episode of intestinal inflammation. Psychological assessment was performed immediately after infection and more than 6 months before IBS symptoms became evident (data from [37]).

While the basic concept of visceral hyperalgesia in post-inflammatory IBS points towards a physiological mechanism which generates the clinical symptoms and marks the well-known psychological characteristics as secondary events, the latter finding calls into attention that psychological traits may well be among the factors which determine who may become a patient with functional bowel disorders, once an organic disease affects the body. Whether this may be a genetic determination or a previously acquired "susceptibility" has to be elucidated in the future.

References

1. Ritchie J. Pain from distension of the pelvic colon by inflating a balloon in the irritable colon syndrome. *Gut* 1973; 14: 125-32.
2. McKee DP, Quigley EM. Intestinal motility in irritable bowel syndrome: is IBS a motility disorder? Part 1. Definition of IBS and colonic motility. *Dig Dis Sci* 1993; 38: 1761-72.
3. McKee DP, Quigley EM. Intestinal motility in irritable bowel syndrome: is IBS a motility disorder? Part 2. Motility of the small bowel, esophagus, stomach and gallbladder. *Dig Dis Sci* 1993; 38: 1773-82.
4. Osterberg E, Blomquist L, Krakau I, Weinryb RM, Asberg M, Hultcrantz R. A population study on irritable bowel syndrome and mental health. *Scand J Gastroenterol* 2000; 35: 264-8.
5. Monnikes H, Tebbe JJ, Hildebrandt M, Arck P, Osmanoglou E, Rose M, Klapp B, Wiedenmann B, Heymann-Monnikes I. Role of stress in functional gastrointestinal disorders. Evidence for stress-induced alterations in gastrointestinal motility and sensitivity. *Dig Dis* 2001; 19: 201-11.
6. Camilleri MD, Choi MG. Review article: irritable bowel syndrome. *Aliment Pharmacol Ther* 1997; 11: 3-15.
7. Thompson WG, Doteval G, Drossman D, Heaton KW, Kruis W. Irritable bowel syndrome: guidelines for the diagnosis. *Gastroenterol Int* 1989; 2: 92-5.
8. Manning AP, Thompson WG, Heaton KW, Morris AF. Towards a positive diagnosis of the irritable bowel syndrome. *Br Med J* 1978: 653-4.
9. Whitehead WE, Engel BT, Schuster MM. Irritable bowel syndrome: physiological and psychological differences between diarrhea-predominant and constipation-predominant patients. *Dis Sci* 1980; 25: 404-13.
10. Whitehead WE, Holtkoetter B, Enck P, Hoelzl R, Holmes KD, Anthony J, Shabsin HS, Schuster MM. Tolerance for rectosigmoid distention in irritable bowel syndrome. *Gastroenterology* 1990; 98: 1187-92.
11. Richter JE, Barish CF, Castell DO. Abnormal sensory perception in patients with esophageal chest pain. *Gastroenterology* 1986; 91: 845-52.
12. Tougas G, Spaziani R, Hollerbach S, Djuric V, Pang C, Upton AR, Fallen EL, Kamath MV. Cardiac autonomic function and oesophageal acid sensitivity in patients with non-cardiac chest pain. *Gut* 2001; 49: 706-12.
13. Mearin F, Cucala M, Azpiroz F, Malagelada JR. The origin of symptoms on the brain-gut axis in functional dyspepsia. *Gastroenterology* 1991; 101: 999-1006.
14. Bradette M, Delvaux M, Staumont G, Fioramonti J, Bueno L, Frexinos J. Evaluation of colonic sensory thresholds in IBS patients using a barostat. Definition of optimal conditions and comparison with healthy subjects. *Dig Dis Sci* 1994; 39: 449-57.
15. Drossman D, *et al.* Rome II: *The functional gastrointestinal disorders*, 2nd ed. Allen Press, Lawrence, 2000: 483-532.
16. Isgar B, Harman M, Kaye MD, Whorwell PJ. Symptoms of irritable bowel syndrome in ulcerative colitis in remission. *Gut* 1998; 24: 190-2.
17. O'Sullivan M, Clayton N, Breslin NP, Harman I, Buntra C, McLaren A, O'Morain CA. Increased mast cells in the irritable bowel syndrome. *Neurogastro* 2000; 12: 449-57.
18. Park CH, Joo YE, Choi SK, Rew JS, Kim SJ, Lee MC. Colonic mast cells in irritable bowel syndrome. *Gastroenterology* 2002; 122: A-552.
19. Chadwick VS, Chen W, Shu D, Paulus B, Bethwaite P, Tie A, Wilson I. Activation of the mucosal immune system in irritable bowel syndrome. *Gastroenterology* 2002; 122: 1778-83.
20. Simren M, Ringström G, Stotzer PO, Abrahamsson H, Björnsson ES. Abnormal levels of neuropeptide Y and peptide YY in colon in the irritable bowel syndrome (IBS). *Gastroenterology* 2001; 120: A753f.

21. Spiller RC, Jenkins D, Thornley JP, Hebden JM, Wright T, Skinner M, Neal KR. Increased rectal mucosal enteroendocrine cells, T lymphocytes, and increased gut permeability following acture Campylobacter enteritis and in post-desynteric irritable bowel syndrome. *Gut* 2000; 47: 804-11.
22. Chang L, Anton P, Reinholdt J, Taing P, Mayer E. Decreased mucosal cytokines in diarrhea-predominant IBS. *Gastroenterology* 2002; 122: A-552.
23. Munakata J, Naliboff B, Harraf F, Kodner A, Lembo T, Chang L, Silverman DH, Mayer EA. Repetitive sigmoid stimulation induces rectal hyperalgesia in patients with irritable bowel syndrome. *Gastroenterology* 1997; 112: 55-63.
24. Sarkar S, Hobson AR, Furlong PL, Woolf CJ, Thompson DG, Aziz Q. Central neural mechanism mediating human visceral hypersensitivity. *Am J Physiol* 2001; 281: G 1196-202.
25. Kern MK, Birn RM, Jaradeh S, Jesmanowicz A, Cox RW, Hyde JS, Shaker R. Identification and characterization of cerebral cortical response to esophageal mucosal acid exposure and distension. *Gastroenterology* 1998; 115: 1353-62.
26. Sato K, Leposavic R, Publicover NG, Sanders KM, Gerthoffer WT. Sensitization of the contractile system of canine colonic smooth muscle by agonists and phorbol ester. *J Physiol* 1994; 481: 677-88.
27. Mayer E, Raybould HE. Role of visceral afferent mechanisms in functional bowel disorders. *Gastroenterology* 1990; 99: 1688-704.
28. Bernstein CN, Niazi N, Robert M, Mertz H, Kodner A, Munakata J, Naliboff B, Mayer EA. Rectal afferent function in patients with inflammatory and functional intestinal disorders. *Pain* 1996; 66: 151-61.
29. Silverman DHS, Munakata JA, Ennes H, Madelkern MA, Hon CK, Mayer EA, Regional cerebral activity in normal and pathological perception of visceral pain. *Gastroenterology* 1997; 112: 64-72.
30. Mertz H, Morgan V, Tanner G, Pickens D, Price R, Shyr Yu, Kessler R. Regional cerebral activation in irritable bowel syndrome and control subjects with painful and nonpainful rectal distention. *Gastroenterology* 2000; 118: 842-8.
31. Naliboff BD, Derbyshire SW, Munakata J, Berman S, Mandelkern M, Chang L, Mayer EA. Cerebral activation in patients with irritable bowel syndrome and control subjects during rectosigmoid stimulation. *Psychosom Med* 2001; 63: 365-75.
32. Bonaz B, Baciu M, Papillon E, Bost R, Gueddah N, Le Bas JF, Fournet J, Segebarth C. Central processing of rectal pain in patients with irritable bowel syndrome: an fMRI study. *Am J Gastroenterol* 2002; 97: 654-61.
33. Crowell MD, Enck P. Brain-gut interactions in visceral sensation and perception. In: Schuster MM, Crowell MD, Koch K, eds. *Schuster Atlas of Gastrointestinal Motility*, 2nd ed. Hamilton/London: BC Decker, 2002: 43-55.
34. Nour S, Svarer C, Kristensen JKI, Paulson OB, Law I. Cerebral activation during micturition in normal men. *Brain* 2000; 123: 781-9.
35. Chaudhary NA, Truelove SC. Human colonic motility: a comparative study of normal subjects, patients with ulcerative colitis, and patients with irritable bowel syndrom. I. Resting patterns of motility. *Gastroenterology* 1961; 40: 1-17.
36. McKendrick MW, Read NW. Irritable bowel syndrome – post salmonella infection. *J Infect* 1994; 29: 1-3.
37. Gwee KA, Graham JC, McKendrick MW, Collins SM, Marshall JS, Walters SJ, Read NW. Psychometric scores and persistence of irritable bowel after infectious diarrhoea. *Lancet* 1996; 347: 150-3.
38. Neal KR, Hebden J, Spiller R. Prevalence of gastrointestinal symptoms six months after bacterial gastroenteritis and risk factors for development of the irritable bowel syndrome: postal survey of patients. *Br Med J* 1997; 314: 779-82.
39. Sarkar S, Aziz Q, Woolf CJ, Hobson AR, Thompson DG. Contribution of central sensitization to the development of non-cardiac chest pain. *Lancet* 2000; 356: 1127-8.

40. Camilleri M, Chey WY, Mayer EA, Northcutt AR, Heath A, Dukes GE, McSorley D, Mangel AM. A randomized controlled clinical trial of the serotonin type 3 receptor antagonist alosetron in women with diarrhea-predominant irritable bowel syndrome. *Arch Intern Med* 2001; 161: 1733-40.
41. Muller-Lissner SA, Fumagalli I, Bardhan KD, Pace F, Pecher E, Nault B, Ruegg P. Tegaserod, a 5-HT (4) receptor partial agonist, relieves symptoms in irritable bowel syndrome patients with abdominal pain, bloating and constipation. *Aliment Pharmacol Ther* 2001; 15: 1655-66.
42. Schikowski A, Thewißen, Mathis C, Ross HG, Enck P. Serotonin type-4 receptors modulate the sensitivity of rectospinal mechanoreceptive afferents in cats. *Neurogastroenterology* 2002; 14: 221-7.
43. Camilleri M. Therapeutic approach to the patient with irritable bowel syndrome. *Am J Med* 1999; 107: 27S-32S.
44. Creed F, Guthrie E. Psychological treatments of the irritable bowel syndrome: a review. *Gut* 1998; 30: 1601-9.

Irritable bowel syndrome: new drugs and therapeutic horizons

Michael J.G. Farthing

Faculty of Medicine, University of Glasgow, United Kingdom

Abstract

There is currently no truly effective therapy for irritable bowel syndrome. The standard approach to date has been to use symptom-directed treatments for diarrhoea, constipation and pain. New drug development has focused predominantly on agents that modify the effects of 5-HT in the gut. $5\text{-}HT_3$ receptor antagonists have been developed for patients with diarrhoea-predominant IBS and have been shown to have some efficacy in women. Unfortunately further development has been hindered by their propensity to cause ischaemic colitis. $5\text{-}HT_4$ receptor agonists are also under evaluation in patients with constipation-predominant IBS. Efficacy has been demonstrated but there are concerns that therapeutic gain may not be sufficient. The observation that IBS may follow an intestinal infection and that sub-clinical inflammation may be present in the colon has prompted a trial of corticosteroid therapy. Unfortunately this did not show clinical efficacy. There is also interest in the possibility that a disturbance of bowel flora might be important promoting trials of antibiotics and probiotics. Basic research continues into single receptor agents particularly CCK1 receptors, tachykinins and other novel neuronal receptors.

Introduction

It may be argued that despite three decades of intense investigation into the pathophysiology of the irritable bowel syndrome (IBS), the management options with respect to pharmacotherapy remain largely unchanged. Even the apparent growth area of the 5-hydroxytryptamine (5-HT) drugs, it is probable that their efficacy at best can only be regarded as modest and may, in a small number of individuals, actually be dangerous. So what has gone wrong? There is clearly no simple answer but it may be partly due to an underlying incompatibility between the desired outcomes of the various stakeholders.

The IBS sufferer

Those with IBS want to understand their symptoms, be certain that they do not have a serious disease that requires specific treatment and gain access to one or more simple remedies that will relieve symptoms rapidly and ideally cure the condition permanently. This for some may mean a drug, a "silver bullet" but for others this may be a full explanation of current concepts behind the pathophysiology of symptom production together with some simple dietary and other lifestyle interventions. For others, in whom there is an underlying affective disorder or stressful life event, some form of psychotherapy or psychotrophic medication may be equally acceptable. For most IBS sufferers, the relief of no longer having to be force fed wheat fibre comes as a great relief!

The doctor

Doctors crave effective pharmacotherapy as avidly as IBS sufferers do. Indeed many clinician scientists have sustained themselves intellectually during the last two decades by indulging in in-depth clinical or laboratory investigations into IBS pathophysiology. Unfortunately scientific endeavour during the past 30 years has not identified the "key defect" in IBS but has thrown up endless pathophysiologic pathways for the therapeutician to consider. In the beginning IBS was a motility disorder. If you were constipated you got fibre or a laxative and if you had diarrhoea you got an anti-diarrhoeal drug. If you had pain you received an anti-spasmodic. But now there are endless, additional theoretical possibilities each with a myriad of potential drug targets. Thus, clinicians have been tantalised by the expanding science of IBS pathogenesis and the brain-gut axis but remain frustrated by the continuing lack of effective new therapies.

The drug developer

IBS has been viewed as a highly fertile area for drug development. In 1999 the financial consultants Lehman Brothers published a detailed market analysis with predictions extending beyond 2007 in which they stated "there is no satisfactory treatment for IBS at present, and most of the drugs used are over a decade old. However, over the next few years we will see the launch of several new products with a potential to transform this stagnant market driving it from a $500 million in 1998 to nearly $3 billion by 2007". The main potential players in this analysis were the 5-HT drugs alosetron, cilansetron, piboserod and tegaserod *(Figure 1)*. However, following the recognition that alosetron is associated with ischaemic colitis the drug was voluntarily withdrawn from the US market and to date there has been no attempt to seek a licence worldwide. Other 5-HT drugs may also be in a precarious position not only because of potential adverse effects but also because of questions relating to efficacy and the magnitude of the therapeutic gain over placebo. A fundamental question remains as to whether any drug directed towards a single receptor would be able to rectify the consortium of intestinal and extra-intestinal symptoms that together constitute IBS. It will be interesting to watch how the industry deals with the current situation in which enormous investment has been made in this therapeutic area but as yet no new agent has arrived in the clinic. How long will this continue to be an affordable strategy?

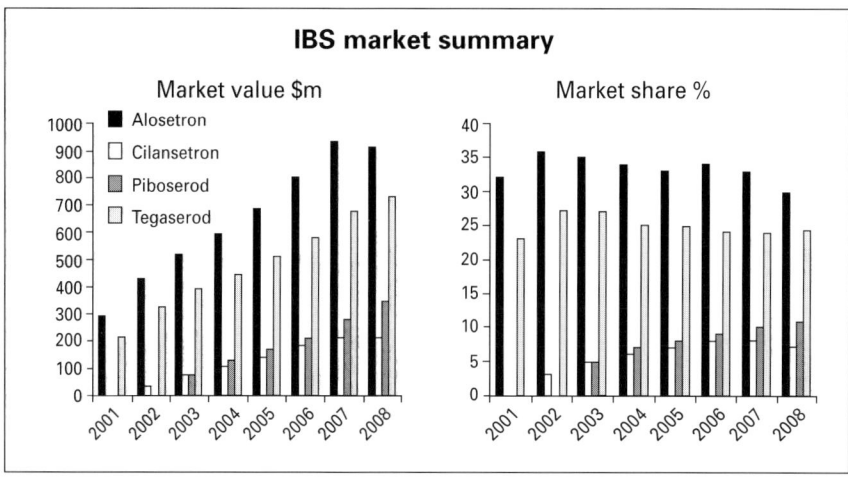

Figure 1. Financial predictions for market value and market share for new 5-HT drugs currently under development. From Lehman Brothers, 1999.

Limitations of current standard therapy

In 1988 Klein published a detailed and in many ways a devastating analysis of randomised controlled trials in IBS [1]. He concluded that the majority of trials of therapeutic agents in IBS were flawed and that none of the agents considered in his review could be regarded as effective in the treatment of IBS. Almost a decade later the American Gastroenterological Association published *A technical review of practice guideline development on IBS*, which included a consensus position on pharmacotherapy in IBS [2]. It acknowledged the poor quality of data on which management decisions were based. More recently Akehurst and Kaltenthaler have again assessed randomised, controlled trials examining the clinical effectiveness of interventions for IBS for 1987-1998 [3]. Forty-five randomised controlled trials were identified but of these only six fulfilled the important three quality criteria, namely, adequate description of randomisation, double blinding and description of withdrawals and dropouts. Thus, it would appear that up to 1998 little progress had been made in improving the quality of clinical evaluation of new treatments in IBS and thus the same concerns that Klein raised in 1988 about standard IBS therapy remain.

Since 1998 there has been a major improvement in the quality of randomised controlled trials for new drugs in IBS, notably those involving the 5-HT drugs. These studies have almost invariably used internationally approved diagnostic criteria, are double-blinded and placebo-controlled and the outcome measures have been clearly defined. There is still debate as to whether global improvement scores should receive more credence than relief of pain and other individual symptoms.

Despite the shortcomings of many of the clinical trials of IBS therapy there is evidence to suggest that some of the time honoured, standard therapies for IBS do have a part to play in management, although for many treatment options this may be limited. Drug therapy for IBS can be considered in two categories: (i) treatments that are aimed predominantly at the gut and based on specific dominant symptoms, so called *end-organ therapy* and (ii) treatment that is aimed at relieving an associated affective disorder or modifying pain pathways in the CNS, namely *central therapy*.

End-organ therapy

Standard agents that are considered to act locally in the gut are shown in *Table I*.

Table I. Standard symptom directed therapy for the irritable bowel syndrome

End-organ therapy	
• Diarrhoea-predominant	Loperamide
	Diphenoxylate
• Constipation-predominant	Increase fibre in diet
	Soluble fibre supplement
	Osmotic laxative (lactulose, magnesium sulphate)
• Pain-predominant	Anticholinergic agents
	Smooth muscle relaxants
	Tricyclic antidepressant
Central therapy	
• Diarrhoea-predominant	Tricyclic antidepressant
• Constipation-predominant	Specific serotonin reuptake inhibitor
• Pain-predominant	Tricyclic antidepressant

Bulking agents do appear to be effective in relieving constipation in some patients with IBS [4]. Recent work however indicates that wheat fibre can exacerbate abdominal pain and bloating which can be minimised if a soluble fibre supplement such as psyllium (ispaghula husk) is used. Anti-diarrhoeal drugs notably loperamide can reduce bowel frequency and improve stool consistency in some patients with diarrhoea-predominant IBS [5].

Abdominal pain in IBS is traditionally treated with drugs which reduce gut spasm such as anti-cholinergics and smooth muscle relaxants. Klein heavily criticised trials performed with this class of drug and concluded from the available studies at that time that there was "no convincing evidence that anti-spasmodic agents are of value" [1]. Since his review further studies have been performed; Poynard *et al.* subjected 26 of these studies which fulfil predetermined inclusion criteria to a meta-analysis [6]. They concluded from this review that five drugs (cimetropium bromide, pinaverium bromide, trimebutine, octilium bromide and mebeverine) have clinical efficacy in IBS. Smooth muscle relaxants significantly improved pain and overall well-being, although they had no effect on abdominal distension. Poynard *et al.* have subsequently carried out a further meta-analysis of smooth muscle relaxants in IBS when 23 randomised clinical trials were selected [7]. Again the meta-analysis favoured the active therapy group with 56% experiencing global improvement in the myorelaxant group compared to 38% in the placebo group. Improvement in pain, however, was less impressive with 53% in the myorelaxant group *versus* 41% in the placebo, thereby producing a therapeutic gain of only 12%.

Central therapy

Central therapy has been considered a reasonable approach to treating some patients with IBS because of an associated affective disorder in a sub-group of patients seeking medical advice. Early clinical trials of antidepressants in IBS however produced inconsistent results although the design and analysis of these studies have been severely criticised [1, 3]. Antidepressants are however clearly effective in depression and there is no reason to believe that depressed patients with IBS would not benefit from their use. The effects of antidepressant drugs on pain threshold are well recognised particularly for the tricyclic antidepressant drugs. Many physicians therefore seriously consider using an antidepressant when pain is an over-riding component of the syndrome.

Our work has confirmed that antidepressants affect gut transit and motility; the tricyclics tend to slow transit while the specific serotonin reuptake inhibitors such as paroxetine tend to produce more rapid transit particularly in the small intestine [8, 9]. These observations should be taken into account when considering the use of these drugs in IBS patients with depression or pain. For patients who are reluctant to take psychotropic medication, there are clinical trials that have shown the therapeutic efficacy of psychotherapy, cognitive therapy and hypnotherapy in IBS [10-13].

The therapeutic challenge of IBS

The consortium of symptoms that include abdominal pain and alterations in the pattern of defaecation, which might in some patients be bowel frequency, in others constipation and in others a combination of the two, presents a formidable challenge to any new therapeutic agents. The complexity is further increased by the common occurrence of other symptoms including abdominal bloating, visible abdominal distension, the feeling of incomplete evacuation and the passage of increased amounts of mucus [14]. Patients with IBS may also complain of symptoms in other parts of the body including urinary symptoms, dyspareunia and fatigue [15]. In addition, IBS can be part of a broad spectrum of functional disorders both within the gastrointestinal tract such as functional dyspepsia, and also with apparently unrelated conditions such as chronic fatigue syndrome, fibromyalgia, temperomandibular joint disorder and chronic pelvic pain [16]. Multivariate analysis suggests that these are distinct disorders and not manifestations of a single somatisation disorder. The close co-morbid association would indicate that there is a common feature important for their expression which at this point would most likely be psychological. This would be supported by the fact that 40-60% of patients with IBS who seek medical advice have psychological symptoms of depression or anxiety, or both.

From this diverse symptomatology it seems unlikely that a single medication can reliably treat all aspects of the syndrome, but it is important to establish therapeutic goals both for clinical trials and for the case management of individuals. Reduction in pain scores, normalisation of bowel habit and global scores of overall well-being are traditionally used, although the global score may be assuming supremacy because of the diversity of symptomatology and the frequency with which symptoms can fluctuate during the trial period. The placebo response rate averages about 40-50% in IBS, which is almost certainly due to the power of reassurance and the non-specific therapeutic effects of entering patients into clinical trials.

Rationale for new drug development in IBS

Models to explain symptom production in IBS have evolved over the last three decades. The tide has ebbed and flowed between the role of end-organ dysfunction and the relative importance of disorders of central control and perception; currently an integrated model is favoured which acknowledges the presence of the brain-gut axis. Since there is no single pathophysiological marker of IBS it seems likely that a complex model which takes into account both central and peripheral factors is the only rational way to proceed until the pathogenesis is more clearly defined [17].

There is now a robust and comprehensive model for a centrally driven pathogenesis of IBS *(Figure 2)* based on the concept of enhanced responsiveness of central stress circuits, the *emotional motor system*. This model can explain many of the features of IBS including disorders of gastrointestinal motility, visceral hypersensitivity, overlap with other functional disorders and co-morbidity with affective disorders and other non-gastrointestinal symptoms [18].

An alternative model is to consider IBS as a primary end-organ disorder which secondarily drives the central manifestations *(Figure 3)*. There is now increasing evidence to suggest that neuroimmune interactions in the gut may play a crucial role in producing end-organ dysfunction particularly with respect to altered motility and visceral sensation [17]. This model proposes that physical stresses in the gut lumen such as an infective agent or an antigen result in changes in the gut immune system involving T lymphocytes and mast cells and also in the number and reactivity of neuroendocrine cells such as enterochromaffin cells. This model has been supported by the now compelling evidence that IBS symptoms can follow an intestinal infection [19-23]. In patients with post-infective IBS, increased numbers of T lymphocytes have been demonstrated in the lamina propria [20] and increased expression of IL-1β mRNA [24]. In addition, enterochromaffin cell numbers have been shown to increase in the colon [25, 26]. Even without persisting abnormalities of gut immune function it is possible that reprogramming of the enteric nervous system following an inflammatory or infective insult might contribute to continuing disordered motility and visceral hypersensitivity. It has been suggested that the functional disturbances sometimes observed in patients with inflammatory bowel disease in remission might be due to a similar persisting neuroimmune dysfunction. It is well known that in inflammatory bowel disease the presence of inflammation can alter anorectal and colonic motility and increase rectal sensitivity which reverses towards normal following treatment [27].

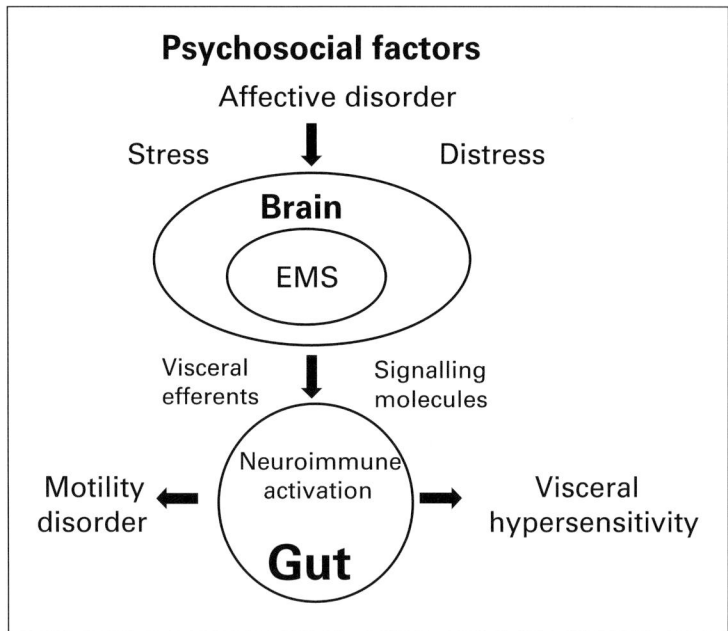

Figure 2. A "central" model to explain pathophysiology and symptom production in IBS. This model proposes that the primary drivers are psychological factors (stress, distress, affective disdorder) which through neural and/or neuroimmune mechanisms result in disturbance of motor and sensory function in the gut.

End-organ neuroimmune dysfunction does not exclude an integrated model. It is well established that psychological stress can promote mast cell degranulation in the gut and can also affect other components of the gut immune system. There is also evidence that immune products released in the gut can act as central signalers through the vagus.

Thus, a complex integrated model of IBS, which incorporates a central component and end-organ dysfunction, appears at present to be the most viable approach to new drug development [17]. The psychosocial stress pathways involving corticotrophin releasing factor (CRF) and the neurotransmitters involved in affective disorders particularly 5-HT and noradrenaline are important potential therapeutic targets for the future. Similarly, the increasingly prominent role of 5-HT in the gut and its possible involvement in both disordered motility and visceral hypersensitivity has already opened up a major new initiative in drug development. The possibility that neuroimmune dysfunction might also become a target for new drug development remains an interesting but speculative option.

New drugs under development for IBS

Drug developers in the field of IBS have explored a number of potential therapeutic targets but by far the most advanced area of research is that of drugs that modify 5-HT in the

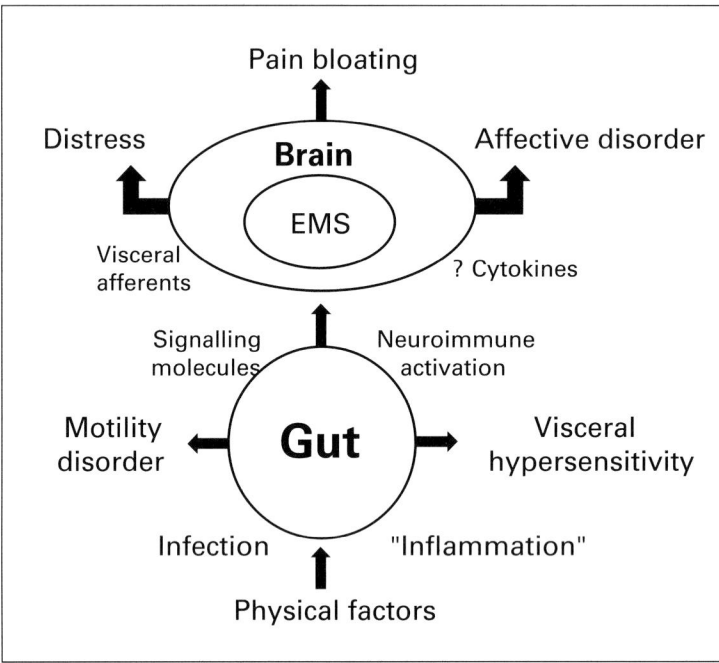

Figure 3. An "end-organ" model to explain the pathophysiology and symptom production in IBS. It proposes that there is a primary disturbance in the gut such as that triggered by an intestinal infection. This might result in neuroimmune activation in the gut with resulting disturbance of motor and sensory function. There may also be more distant effects in the brain mediated by visceral afferent and possible other signalling molecules such as cytokines.

gut, namely 5-HT antagonists and 5-HT agonists [28-30]. Other potential areas under consideration include kappa opioid agonists, and other receptors on sensory neurones including cholecystokinin CCK1 receptors, glutamate receptors and tachykinin receptors. More recently there have been attempts to modify a possible inflammatory component in IBS including attempts to modify the bowel flora either with antibiotics or probiotics and by using anti-inflammatory drugs such as corticosteroids.

5-hydroxytryptamine modifying drugs

5-HT is found widely in the alimentary tract and the central nervous system; 90% of the 5-HT in the body is found in the gut, most of which is in enterochromaffin cells with only 5% in enteric neurones where it is now considered to act as a neurotransmitter [30]. 5-HT has an important physiological role during a number of normal events in the gut, particularly the motor and secretory responses to the ingestion of food. 5-HT is released from enterochromaffin cells in response to a number of stimuli including touch, changes in pressure, acid and food. As a mucosal signalling module 5-HT activates intrinsic nerves with involvement in peristalsis and intestinal secretion, it also activates extrinsic nerves typically following release by chemotherapeutic agents when it can produce nausea and vomitting, bloating and pain [31]. In addition there is now increasing evidence that 5-HT may be involved in the pathogenesis of diarrhoea during some intestinal infections, particularly cholera and may contribute to symptom production in intestinal obstruction. The relevance of 5-HT to IBS relates to several lines of evidence. There are experimental data to suggest that patients with diarrhoea-predominant IBS release more 5-HT than healthy volunteers following a standard meal [32, 33]. Enterochromaffin cell numbers are increased in the colon in patients with IBS [26] and also in patients with post-dysenteric IBS [25]. It is known that 5-HT sensitises visceral nerves and the enteric nervous system and thus it seems entirely rational to attempt to modulate the effects of 5-HT with a view to improving both the motor and sensory symptoms in this condition.

The major receptor targets that have been explored are the $5\text{-}HT_3$ and $5\text{-}HT_4$ receptors [34, 35].

5-HT3 receptor antagonists

Drugs such as ondansetron and granisetron were a major advance in the treatment of chemotherapy-induced emesis. It is thought that these drugs antagonise the effects of 5-HT both in the visceral afferent nerves from the gut and also in the brain stem. It was postulated therefore that this class of drug might be useful in IBS by reducing sensitisation, reducing pain and retarding transit accepting the possibility that they might cause constipation. $5\text{-}HT_3$ receptor antagonists reduce the effects of nociceptive stimuli in the skin and in gut model systems. Some $5\text{-}HT_3$ receptor antagonists such as granisetron and alosetron reduce rectal hypersensitivity in IBS patients although there are some inconsistencies in the literature possibly relating to experimental technique and subject selection [36-39]. Alosetron and cilansetron have been subjected to evaluation by randomised controlled trials and both are considered to have some efficacy in patients with diarrhoea-predominant IBS.

In the major alosetron study [40] the primary end point was adequate relief of IBS pain and discomfort for at least two weeks per month. Patients who achieved this end-point were regarded as responders. Since a previous study had shown that men did not improve on alosetron, the study was restricted to women; 41% of patients on alosetron reported adequate relief of pain for all three months of the study compared to 29% on placebo. This amounts to a 12% therapeutic gain over placebo. Alosetron also decreased urgency and stool frequency and increased stool consistency. There were some problems with the study in that 30% of the alosetron group experienced constipation (only 3% in placebo group) which was the major reason for the 24% drop out rate in the alosetron group. Actual pain scores were not reported in the paper but an analysis was performed by the Public Citizens Research Group and published in the correspondence columns of the *Lancet* which showed there was no difference in absolute pain and discomfort scores in alosetron and placebo treated patients.

Several other studies confirmed that alosetron had some efficacy in diarrhoea-predominant IBS in women [41]. The drug received a product licence in the USA in February 2000 but during the ensuing months it became clear that there were an increasing number of reports of ischaemic colitis and severe constipation, many of which required hospitalisation and included five deaths. The manufacturer withdrew the drug in November 2000. Other 5-HT$_3$ receptor antagonists are also under development, cilansetron being the most advanced in the process [42]. Unfortunately one case of ischaemic colitis has already been reported with cilansetron and thus it seems likely that this will be shown to be a class-specific adverse effect. The precise mechanism as to how alosetron causes ischaemic colitis has not been clearly established although 5-HT is well-known to be a vasodilator and dose-dependent inhibition of 5-HT induced cutaneous erythema is a well-established bioassay for 5-HT$_3$ receptor antagonists.

5-HT4 receptor agonists

The rationale for the development of this class of drug for IBS was based on anticipated effects on the gut motility in that they would be expected to be prokinetic and thereby reduce constipation but in addition it was anticipated that they might have an independent effect in reducing visceral hypersensitivity. 5-HT$_4$ receptors are thought to be located on cholinergic interneurones and motor neurones. 5-HT$_4$ agonists inhibit slow depolarization responses in myenteric neurones imitating the action of 5-HT. 5-HT$_4$ receptors have also been identified on smooth muscle and enterocytes. 5-HT$_4$ agonists are prokinetic and may also modulate sensory pathways [34].

The drug in this class that is most advanced along the development pathway is tegaserod, an aminoguanidine indole derivative of 5-HT which acts as a partial 5-HT$_4$ receptor agonist. Tegaserod stimulates peristalsis, increases small intestinal and colonic motility and speeds up intestinal transit [43].

There have been three major randomized controlled trials of tegaserod compared to placebo in patients with constipation predominant IBS [43-45]. These studies predominantly involved women (83-87%) and compared 4 mg and 12 mg doses with placebo. The endpoints were global improvement, and improvement in abdominal pain, bowel frequency and stool consistency. In the first study (B301), there was significant improvement in abdominal pain at both doses although the therapeutic gain was only 9% and 8% respectively. In the second study (B307), there was no difference between tegaserod and placebo at either dose but in the third study (B351) only the 12 mg dose had significant benefit over placebo with a therapeutic gain of 12%. Like alosetron, no therapeutic benefits were demonstrated in males although relatively few men were included in these studies and thus a type 2 error cannot be excluded. Diarrhoea was the major unwanted adverse effect which occurred in 12% of patients. A recent meta-analysis containing a fourth trial confirmed the therapeutic efficacy of tegaserod [46]. Thus although a *statistically* significant benefit has been demonstrated over placebo the question remains as to whether this is a *clinically* significant effect and whether a similar therapeutic gain might be obtained with a simple laxative or soluble fibre.

The relevance of the clinical efficacy of tegaserod has been questioned by the European Agency for Evaluation of Medicinal Products and thus further clinical studies are underway. Similarly the US Food and Drug Administration has raised concerns about the drug and abdominal surgical events particularly because of the effects of tegaserod on gallbladder motility. Thus the future of tegaserod in both the USA and Europe remains uncertain.

Prucalopride is a selective 5-HT$_4$ agonist, is prokinetic and has been shown to improve stool frequency and consistency in patients with constipation. However, concerns have been raised about its safety particularly with respect to carcinogenicity and possible cardiotoxic effects. Currently the clinical development programme has been suspended awaiting the outcome of further testing.

Kappa receptor agonists

An alternative approach to reducing abdominal pain has been the use of opioid κ agonists such as trimebutine and fedotozine. A double-blind, randomized controlled trial has shown that fedotozine can reduce abdominal pain, post-prandial fullness and bloating in patients with non-ulcer dyspepsia. Fedotozine (3.5-30 mg three times daily) was compared with placebo in a randomized, controlled trial during a 6-week period in patients with IBS. Fedotozine 30 mg daily was superior to placebo in relieving abdominal pain and bloating [47]. Although the assessment of bowel function appeared to be inadequate in this study, there were no obvious changes in bowel frequency and stool consistency. Despite the apparent efficacy of fedotozine in IBS, this drug is not being promoted for the treatment of either non-ulcer dyspepsia or IBS on the grounds that its therapeutic advantage is not significantly greater than established drugs.

Somatostatin and its analogues are known to have analgesic effects on somatic and visceral pain. There is limited evidence in humans that this approach might have a role in the management of IBS [48] although it is unlikely that any of the currently available preparations would be appropriate because of potential adverse effects following prolonged use in an otherwise benign disorder.

Modification of the bowel flora

The rationale for attempting to modify the bowel flora emanates from the observation that small bowel bacterial overgrowth may be associated with IBS in some patients [49]. This is counterintuitive for two reasons; published evidence would indicate that small bowel transit in IBS is either decreased or normal [50], but certainly not increased. In addition the diarrhoea associated with bacterial overgrowth is generally accompanied by steatorrhoea which again is not the case in IBS. However in one study using the lactulose hydrogen breath test 157 of 202 IBS patients (78%) were considered to have small bowel bacterial overgrowth; 48% of patients that were satisfactorily treated with antibiotics showed improvement in IBS symptoms such that they no longer met Rome diagnostic criteria [49]. Caution should be exercised in the interpretation of this study since an additional confirmatory assessment of bacterial overgrowth was not made (such as bacterial culture of duodenal fluid, or a bile salt or glucose breath test); the apparent abnormality of the lactulose breath test could merely be due to rapid transit. This would not explain the response to antibiotics but the number of subjects treated was small and it was not a randomized controlled trial. Elemental diet however has been shown to be more effective than antibiotics in normalizing lactulose breath test in IBS [51]. Although it is postulated that this effect is mediated by an effect on distal bowel flora, an effect on transit cannot be excluded.

Anti-inflammatory therapy

There has also been interest in modifying the bowel flora with a view to diminishing the effects of persistent neuro-immune activation in the gut. There have been a number of trials of probiotics in IBS although patient numbers tend to be small and treatment period often less than the accepted ideal of 8-12 weeks. Lactobacillus and bifidobacterium preparations are reported to be effective although there are inconsistencies in published data and some evidence for strain dependency [52, 53]. A recent meta-analysis of 12 clinical trials would support more extensive and rigorous testing although the authors acknowledge the shortcomings of some of the study designs [54].

The use of prednisolone has now been formally trialled in IBS. Thirty-one patients with post-infective IBS were treated with prednisolone 30 mg daily or placebo for three weeks and symptoms evaluated during weeks 3-5 [55]. Changes in mucosal inflammation were assessed in rectal biopsies. Although CD3 lymphocyte counts decreased, there was no improvement in IBS symptoms. There continues to be a major scientific interest in the possibility that persistent, low grade inflammation may be an important determinant of IBS symptoms particularly in post-infective IBS; this study would suggest that, even if this is true, it is not a simple relationship as that found in non-specific inflammatory bowel disease. An alternative explanation might be that the relatively minor abnormalities reported are insufficient to explain the observed abnormalities of gut function in IBS.

Future horizons

The development of new therapies for IBS is at an impasse. Despite new insights into pathophysiology and a major clinical development programme into 5-HT drugs there are no new drugs available for IBS sufferers. Perhaps the manufacturers of the 5-HT drugs have so far been unlucky? The concepts were right but the drugs were not strong enough or late in the day were found to have adverse effects which could not be justified in this relatively mild, non-fatal condition. On the other hand, perhaps the underlying premise was wrong? It may be too simplistic to hope that a disorder with such a complex pathophysiology involving dysfunction of the enteric nervous system, with possibly neuroimmune overtones and the brain gut axis will be resolved by a highly selective agent targeting a single receptor. Understanding the subtle differences between different sub-groups of IBS may provide additional evidence to support this approach but to date it has to be accepted that there are no major therapeutic triumphs.

There is however continuing interest in the single receptor approach with the possibility that 5-HT$_1$ receptor agonists might have a role in IBS because of their known efficacy in functional dyspepsia. In addition the search for anti-nociceptive drugs continues, a particular target being the dorsal horn neurones of the spinal cord. A candidate target might be the N-methyl-D-aspartate (NMDA)-type glutamate receptors located on small diameter pain fibres. Activation of the NMDA receptor causes release of substance P which interacts synergistically with glutamate in the excitation of dorsal horn nociceptive neurones resulting in the production of pain. Other possible candidates include tachykinin and cholecystokinin antagonists.

One might predict, however, that the single receptor approach may not be successful and that many, possibly all, of these candidate targets will not produce affordable drugs of sufficient efficacy. Statistically significant clinical trials of a new IBS drug against placebo do not necessarily mean that a drug will offer a clinically significant benefit. Thompson in his recent review of treatment of IBS made a bold statement: "most irritable bowel syndrome sufferers require no drug" [56]. Perhaps this concept should be actively incorporated more vigorously into future IBS therapeutic strategies.

References

1. Klein KB. Controlled treatment trials in the irritable bowel syndrome: a critique. *Gastroenterology* 1977; 95: 232-41.
2. Drossman DA, Whitehead WE, Camilleri M. Irritable bowel syndrome: a technical review for practice guideline development. *Gastroenterology* 1997; 112: 2120-37.
3. Akehurst R, Kaltenthaler E. Treatment of irritable bowel syndrome: a review of randomised controlled trials. *Gut* 2001; 48: 272-83.
4. Francis CY, Whorwell PJ. Bran and irritable bowel syndrome: time for reappraisal. *Lancet* 1994; 344: 39-40.
5. Efskind PS, Bernklev T, Vatn MH. A double-blind placebo-controlled trial with loperamide in irritable bowel syndrome. *Scand J Gastroenterol* 1996; 31: 463-8.
6. Poynard T, Naveau S, Mory B, et al. Meta-analysis of smooth muscle relaxants in the treatment of irritable bowel syndrome. *Aliment Pharmacol Ther* 1994; 8: 499-510.
7. Poynard T, Regimbeau C, Benhamou Y. Meta-analysis of smooth muscle relaxants in the treatment of irritable bowel syndrome. *Aliment Pharmacol Ther* 2001; 15: 355-61.
8. Gorard DA, Libby GW, Farthing MJG. Effect of a tricyclic anti-depressant on small intestinal motility in health and in diarrhea-predominant irritable bowel syndrome. *Dig Dis Sci* 1995; 40: 86-95.
9. Gorard DA. Libby GW, Farthing MJG. 5 hydroxytryptamine and human small intestinal motility: effect of inhibiting 5-hydroxytryptamine uptake. *Gut* 1994; 34: 496-500.
10. Whorwell PJ, Prior A, Feragher EB. Control trial of hypnotherapy in the treatment of severe refractory irritable bowel syndrome. *Lancet* 1984; ii: 1232-4.
11. Whorwell PJ, Prior A, Colgan SM. Hypnotherapy in severe irritable bowel syndrome; further experience. *Gut* 1987; 28: 423-5.
12. Guthrie E. A brief psychotherapy with patients with refractory IBS. *Br J Psychother* 1991; 8: 175-88.
13. Guthrie E, Creed F. The difficult patient: treating the mind and the gut. *Eur J Gastroenterol Hepatol* 1994; 6: 489-94.
14. Farthing MJG. Irritable bowel, irritable body, irritable brain? *Br Med J* 1995; 310: 171-5.

15. Whorwell PJ, McCallum M, Creed FH, *et al.* Non-colonic features of irritable bowel syndrome. *Gut* 1986; 27: 37-40.
16. Gomborone JE, Gorard DA, Dewsnap PA, *et al.* Prevalence of irritable bowel syndrome in chronic fatigue. *J Roy Coll Phys* 1996; 30: 512-3.
17. Mayer EA, Collin SM. Evolving pathophysiologic models of functional gastrointestinal disorders. *Gastroenterology* 2002; 122: 2032-48.
18. Mayer EA. The neurobiology of stress and gastrointestinal disease. *Gut* 2000; 47: 861-9.
19. Gwee KA, Graham JC, McKendrick MW, *et al.* Psychometric scores and persistence of irritable bowel after infectious diarrhoea. *Lancet* 1996: 347: 150-3.
20. Gwee KA, Leong YL, Graham C, *et al.* The role of psychological and biological factors in post infective gut dysfunction. *Gut* 1999; 44: 400-6.
21. McKendrick MW, Read NW. Irritable bowel syndrome - post *Salmonella* infection. *J Infect* 1994; 29: 1-3.
22. McKendrick MW. Post *Salmonella* irritable bowel syndrome – 5 year review. *J Infect* 1996; 32: 170-1.
23. Neal KR, Hebden J, Spiller R. Prevalence of gastrointestinal symptoms six months after bacterial gastroenteritis and risk factors for development of the irritable bowel syndrome; postal survey of patients. *Br Med J* 1997; 314: 779-82.
24. Gwee KA, Collins SM, Marshall JS, Underwood JE, Moochala SM, Read NW. Evidence of inflammatory pathogenesis in post-infectious irritable bowel syndrome. *Gastroenterology* 1998; 114: 758.
25. Spiller RC, Jenkins D, Thornley JP, Hebden JM, Wright T, Skinner M, Neal KR. Increased rectal mucosal enteroendocrine cells, T-lymphocytes and increased gut permeability following acute *Campylobacter* enteritis and in post-dysenteric irritable bowel syndrome. *Gut* 2000; 47: 804-11.
26. Bose M, Nickols C, Feakins R, Greenwald, Farthing MJG. A comparison of 5-hydroxytryptamine staining in enterochronomaffin cells between irritable bowel syndrome and other gastrointestinal disorders. *Gut* 2000; 47 (Suppl. III): A 210.
27. Farthing MJG, Lennard-Jones JE. Sensibility of the rectum to distension and the anorectal distension reflex in ulcerative colitis. *Gut* 1978; 19: 64-9.
28. Farthing MJG. 5-hydroxytryptamine and 5-hydroxytryptamine-3 receptor antagonists. *Scand J Gastroenterol* 1991; 26: 92-100.
29. Farthing MJG. New drugs in the management of the irritable bowel syndrome. *Drugs* 1998; 56: 11-21.
30. Farthing MJG. Irritable bowel syndrome: new pharmaceutical approaches to treatment. *Bailliere's Clin Gastroenterol* 1999; 13: 461-71.
31. Sanger GJ. 5-hydroxytryptamine and functional bowel disorders. *Neurogastroenterol Motil* 1996; 8: 319-31.
32. Bearcroft CP, Perrett D, Farthing MJG. Post-prandial plasma 5-hydroxytryptamine in diarrhoea predominant irritable bowel syndrome. *Gut* 1998; 42: 42-6.
33. Houghton LA, Whitaker P, Atkinson W, Whorwell PJ, Fricker J, Rimer M, Jaques L, Mills J. Increased platelet stores of 5-hydroxytryptamine (5-HT) in female patients with diarrhoea predominant irritable bowel syndrome (IBS). *Gastroenterology* 2001; (Suppl. 1): A636.
34. Sanger GJ. Different pathophysiological functions of $5-HT_4$ and $5-HT_3$ receptors in small and large intestine. *Curr Res Serotonin* 1998; 3: 99-104.
35. Sanger GJ. Therapeutic applications of $5-HT_4$ receptor agonists and antagonists. In: Eglen RM, ed. *$5-HT_4$ receptors in the brain and periphery*. Springer-Verlag & RG Landes Co, 1998: 213-26.
36. Prior A, Read NW. Reduction of rectal sensitivity and post-prandial motility by granisetron, $5-HT_3$ receptor antagonist, in patients with irritable bowel syndrome. *Aliment Pharmacol Ther* 1993: 175-80.
37. Hammer J, Phillips SF, Talley NJ, *et al.* Effect of a $5-HT_3$ antagonist (ondansetron) on rectal sensitivity and compliance in health and the irritable bowel syndrome. *Aliment Pharmacol Ther* 1993; 7: 543-51.

38. Goldberg PA, Kamm MA, Setti-Carraro P, *et al.* Modification of visceral sensitivity and pain in irritable bowel syndrome by 5-HT$_3$ antagonism (ondansetron). *Digestion* 1996; 57: 478-83.
39. Banner SE, Sanger GJ. Differences between 5-HT3 receptor antagonists in modulation of visceral hypersensitivity. *Br J Pharmacol* 1995; 114: 558-62.
40. Camilleri M, Nortcutt AR, Kong S, Dukes GE, McSorley D, Mangel AW. Efficacy and safety of alosetron in women with irritable bowel syndrome: a randomised, placebo-controlled trial. *Lancet* 2000; 355: 1035-40.
41. Camilleri M, Chey WY, Mayer EA, Northcutt AR, Heath A, Dukes GE, McSorley D, Mangel AM. A randomized controlled clinical trial of the serotonin type 3 receptor antagonist alosetron in women with diarrhea-predominant irritable bowel syndrome. *Arch Intern Med* 2001; 161: 1733-40.
42. Rabasseda X, Leeson P, Silvestre J, Castaner J. Cilansetron. *Drugs of the Future* 1999; 24: 475-82.
43. Camilleri M. Review article: tegaserod. *Aliment Pharmacol Ther* 2001: 15: 277-89.
44. Muller-Lissner SA, Fumagalli I, Bardhan KD, Pace F, Pecher E, Nault B, Ruegg P. Tegaserod, a 5-HT$_4$ receptor partial agonist, relieves symptoms in irritable bowel syndrome patients with abdominal pain, bloating and constipation. *Aliment Pharmacol Ther* 2001; 15: 1655-66.
45. Lefkowitz M. Safety and tolerability of tegaserod in patients with irritable bowel syndrome and diarrhea symptoms. *Am J Gastroenterol* 2002; 97: 1176-81.
46. Schoenfeld P, Chey WD, Drossman D, Kim HM, Thompson WG. Effectiveness and safety of tegaserod in the treatment of irritable bowel syndrome: a meta-analysis of randomized controlled trials. *Gastroenterology* 2002, in press.
47. Dapoigny M, Abitbol JL, Fraitag B. Efficacy of peripheral kappa agonist fedotozine *versus* placebo in treatment of irritable bowel syndrome. *Dig Dis Sci* 1995; 40: 2244-8.
48. Talley NJ, Turner I, Middleton WR. Somatostatin and symptomatic relief of irritable bowel syndrome. *Lancet* 1987; 11: 1114.
49. Pimental M, Chow EJ, Lin HC. Eradication of small intestinal bacterial overgrowth reduces symptoms of irritable bowel syndrome. *Am J Gastroenterol* 2000; 95: 3503-6.
50. Gorard DA, Farthing MJG. Intestinal motor function in irritable bowel syndrome. *Dig Dis Sci* 1994: 12: 72-4.
51. Pimentel M, Bajwa M, Constantino TA, Kong Y, Lin HC. Elemental diet is more effective than antibiotics in normalizing lactulose breath test in IBS. *Gastroenterology* 2002, in press.
52. Niedzielin K. A controlled, double-blind randomized study on the efficacy of Lactobacillus plantarum 299V in patients with irritable bowel syndrome. *Eur J Gastroenterol Hepatol* 2001; 13: 1143-7.
53. Quigley E, O'Mahoney L, McCarthy J, Kelly P, Collins JK, Shanahan F, O'Sullivan G, Kiely B. Probiotics for the irritable bowel syndrome (IBS): a randomized, double-blind, placebo-controlled comparison of Lactobacillus and Bifidobacterium strains. *Gastroenterology* 2002, in press.
54. Hamilton-Miller, JMT. Probiotics in the management of irritable bowel syndrome: a review of clinical trials. *Microb Ecol Health Dis* 2001; 3: 212-6.
55. Dunlop S, Jenkins D, Naesdal J, Borgaonker M, Collins S, Spiller R. Randomised double-blind placebo-controlled trial of prednisolone in post-infectious irritable bowel syndrome (PI-IBS). *Gastroenterology* 2002, in press.
56. Thompson WG. Review article: the treatment of irritable bowel syndrome. *Aliment Pharmacol Ther* 2002; 16: 1395-406.

new approaches to management
of gastrointestinal stromal tumors

Fabio Farinati, Romilda Cardin, Massimo De Giorgio, Simona Gianni

Section of Gastroenterology, Department of Surgical and Gastroenterological Sciences, Padua University, Italy

Abstract

Gastrointestinal stromal tumors (GISTs) are rare mesenchymal tumors, with a poorly understood origin and a wide spectrum of differentiation. They are however characterized by the expression of the transmembrane receptor tyrosine kinase KIT, which is identified as CD117 antigen and is the product of the c-kit proto-oncogene. A malignant behaviour is predicted by tumor size and cytoproliferation rate and, when malignant, tumor spreading beyond organ of origin at the time of diagnosis is frequent. Surgery is the primary treatment modality but, when the tumor is advanced or metastatic, chemotherapy and radiation treatment are lacking any efficacy. The finding that c-kit is upregulated in this kind of tumors has recently suggested new alternative treatment approaches to advanced disease. Imatinib is a new type of tyrosine kinase inhibitor that selectively inhibits various tyrosine kinases and its role in the treatment of GISTs is confirmed by preclinical studies. Recently published clinical data are prompting great enthusiasm with respect to the efficacy and the safety of the drug in the treatment of advanced GISTs.

Epidemiology and pathogenesis

Gastrointestinal stromal tumors (GISTs) are the most frequent mesenchymal tumors of gastrointestinal tract but, despite this, their origin is poorly understood. The cells involved present some similarity to the interstitial cells of Cajal (ICCs), that are supposed to be part of a complex system acting as a pace-maker for the gastrointestinal tract. Beyond that, also the mutations found in the c-kit gene may suggest origin from ICCs and/or multipotential mesenchymal cells that differentiated into ICCs.

The peak of incidence for this tumor is in the adulthood (fifth and sixth decade), and young people under the age of 40 are very rarely involved. There is not a clear-cut gender predilection, although a few studies show a male predominance. The true incidence is not known; but calculations, dating in the eighties, estimated approximately 150 new GISTs per year in the United States [1].

GISTs may present throughout the gastrointestinal tract from as high as in the pharynx to as low as in the anus; the incidence in a single organ being therefore quite low. They have been reported to represent < 1% of malignancies of the esophagus, stomach, colon and rectum. In the small bowel, the diagnosis of stromal tumors account for 20% of the neoplasm when carcinomas and lymphomas have been histologically excluded. The most frequent region involved is stomach (52-70% of the cases), followed by the small intestine (20-25%); while localization of the tumor in other sites such as large bowel, esophagus, peritoneum is quite occasional [2, 3]. Up to two thirds of GISTs are malignant, if we except the esophagus, where virtually all are benign. The risk factors and etiology of GIST remain undetermined.

Pathology

GISTs are not a uniform type of disease from the morphological point of view: they depict a broad spectrum of differentiation ranging from complete differentiated tumors with myoid (*i.e.* leiomyoma or leiomyosarcoma-type), neural (*i.e.* schwannoma-type), or ganglionic plexus phenotypes (*i.e.* ganglioneuroma or plexosarcoma-type) to tumors with incomplete, mixed or totally lacking differentiation. Some tumors present autonomic nervous system resemblance and are consequently classified as gastrointestinal autonomic nervous tumors (GANT). GISTs may show a wide range of size (from millimeters to over 30 cm) [4] and are generally smooth greyish tumors arising within the muscularis propria of the GI tract. They usually present a pseudocapsule, with an endophytic growth that often leads to obstructive events while an exophytic growth is more rarely found.

Cytologically, the tumor cells may present various appearance: spindle-shaped, round (epithelioid), plasmacytoid, mixoid, signet ring, granular or multinucleated, with either benign or malignant cytologic features.

Immunohistochemical features

The expression of transmembrane receptor tyrosine kinase KIT, which is identified as the CD117 antigen and is the product of the c-kit proto-oncogene, is peculiar of GISTs. This is a low molecular weight molecule consisting of only 976 amino acids, with an extracellular domain composed of five immunoglobulin-like regions, a transmembrane domain and an intracellular domain responsible for the kinase activity. The gene product is widely expressed in normal tissues, but activation or gain-of-function mutations in the c-kit gene have been identified in the majority of GISTs.

Beyond that, several additional genetic changes are being discovered including losses in 14q and 22q in both benign and malignant GISTs. For instance, a specific germline mutation in exon 11 has been detected in about 65% of GISTs [5]; this kind of mutation produces an inherited susceptibility to the formation of GISTs, that is autosomic and dominant, with the affected individuals developing diffuse hyperplasia of ICC and multiple GISTs in adulthood [6].

There is no consensus about the immuno-histopathological criteria for categorising an intestinal mesenchymal tumor as a GIST, a reason for the disagreement being related to the choice of monoclonal and polyclonal antibodies, as well as to the differences in the technical parameters used and variable interpretation of the staining results.

The antibodies most commonly used target muscle specific actin, smooth muscle actin (SMA), S100 protein and neurofilament (NF). In this sense, monoclonal and polyclonal antibodies directed at the c-kit gene product expressed on the cell surface (CD117/c-kit) appear to be increasingly helpful in resolving the differential diagnosis between GISTs and other gastrointestinal smooth muscle neoplasms, schwannomas and others. Another sensitive immunohistological marker for GISTs is CD34. This is a 110 kDa transmembrane glycoprotein found on human haematopoietic progenitor cells and vascular endothelium, expressed by a wide variety of tumors and detectable in 50-80% of GISTs. However, CD34 may also be expressed by true smooth muscle cells, and is not therefore a specific marker. CD117 is not expressed in smooth muscle or neural tumors and is consequently quite helpful in the differential diagnosis between GISTs and other gastrointestinal mesenchymal tumors. Recent data on GISTs in the omentum, peritoneum and retroperitoneum has also reinforced the importance of CD117 in making the distinction between GISTs at unusual locations and morphologically comparable mesenchymal tumors at these sites.

Finally CD117 immunostaining, together with mitotic index or evaluation of S-phase fraction, is also gaining a prognostic role in GISTs as documented by several recent studies [7, 8].

Clinical features

Affected patients may be totally asymptomatic, the tumor being an accidental finding, while symptoms are generally variable according with the tumor size and localization. Abdominal pain or bleeding are described as the most frequent symptoms (especially for tumors of stomach or small bowel), due to ulceration (which is also considered, when present, a sign of malignancy). Obstruction, dysphagia, or altered bowel habits could be the first manifestations in the esophagus or rectum. The remaining symptoms may include anorexia, perforation or fever.

When malignancy is present, spreading of the tumor beyond organ of origin at the time of diagnosis is frequent. The developing of hepatic metastases and the presence of local recurrence are the main features of failure of treatment while the tumors locally confined at diagnosis and found incidentally during surgery generally present a benign behaviour.

Endosonographic studies reported a number of features often related to malignancy including: tumor size of > 4 cm, irregular borders, hyper-echogenic foci, and cystic spaces. When two or three of these features are present, a diagnosis of malignancy can be suspected with 80-100% confidence [9].

Carney *et al.* described in 1977 a rare triad ("Carney's triad") of associated tumors: gastric (epithelioid) leiomyosarcoma, functioning extra-adrenal paraganglioma, and pulmonary chondroma. Since that time, they have identified a total of 79 affected patients, the majority of them having only two tumors. The triad represented a chronic and indolent disease; with a survival rate at 20-year follow-up of about 80%. It is very important to stress the idea that these patients must have life-long surveillance, since the triad may develop with a long time interval.

Anatomical site

The anatomical location of GIST is a very important predictive factor, since it is generally accepted that biological behaviour may differ significantly with location.

In the stomach, GISTs usually involve the body region (around 40% of the cases) and more rarely the antrum and pylorus, with the submucosa more frequently affected [10]. Gastric GISTs diameters range from a few millimeters to 15 cm and the most common clinical manifestations are gastrointestinal bleeding, pain, and fatigue or malaise.

Benign duodenal GISTs are usually small and show low cellularity, with spindle cell type, an organoid architecture and less than 2 mitoses/50 high power field (HPF) [11].

Malignant tumors are larger, have more mitoses and are hypercellular and epithelioid. A size larger than 5 cm is, for jejunum and ileum, considered a predictive factor of malignancy.

A rare association of Crohn's disease in the terminal ileum with high-risk GISTs has been described [12].

In the colon, a diameter of less than 2 cm can indicate benignity, and size larger than 5 cm associated with a mitotic rate greater than 5/10 are generally considered as predictors of malignancy.

Prognostic factors

Grading a GIST is not an easy task. Some authors [13] divided GIST into three prognostic groups: benign, borderline and malignant, this being a generally accepted classification. Size, as already reported above, and mitotic rate are the most powerful predictive factors associated with malignant behaviour. In particular, size > 5 cm is described a factor often associated with poor prognosis; however, this is not a completely reliable predictor of biological behaviour since in some instances tumors smaller than 5 cm in size have been shown to metastasize [14]. Mitotic index is a strong predictor of malignancy and of prognosis. However, there is even no consensus on how to express the ratio. A mitotic index ranging from 1 to 5/10 high power fields (HPF) seems to be associated with increased metastatic potential. GISTs can be further subgrouped into low grade (< 10 mitosis/10 HPF) and high grade (> 10 mitosis/10 HPF) lesions. Benign stromal tumors are those with 0-1 mitosis/10 HPF. In a study by Yu et al. [15], low grade tumors (0-1 mitosis/30 HPF) were associated with 5- and 10-year survival rates of 100%, while intermediate grade tumors ($\geq$ 5/30 HPF) were associated with 5- and 10-year survival rates of 12% and 13%, respectively. However, even lesions considered likely to behave in a benign fashion are best regarded as having an uncertain malignant potential, because they may recur many years after initial resection.

Finally, high-grade lesions ($\geq$ 10/10 HPF), in a study with long follow-up, showed a 5- and 10-year survival rate of 5% and 0%, respectively [16].

Management

There is a consensus on the fact that chemotherapy and radiation treatment are lacking any efficacy in GISTs even though no RCT have been performed to evaluate their role. Surgery is the primary treatment modality, the radical treatment being represented by complete and extensive surgical resection. Intra-operative frozen section examination should be performed in order to differentiate stromal tumor from adenocarcinoma and lymphoma, since the diagnosis is often difficult to make preoperatively. When frozen section diagnosis is suggestive of stromal tumor, the treatment should be the one of the malignant diseases. *En bloc* resection should be considered when contiguous organs are involved. Despite complete resection with pathologically confirmed negative margins, the majority of tumors recur (about 70% of gastric tumors and about 60% of small and large bowel) [17], usually with local or peritoneal involvement, often in association with liver metastasis. Extra-abdominal disease in the absence of peritoneal involvement is rare. Although most recurrence occur within 2 years, tumors with low mitotic index may take > 10 years to metastasize, emphasizing the need for a long-term follow-up.

There are few reports describing a survival advantage after resection of abdominal recurrences [18] and the role, if any, of aggressive surgery in the treatment of metastatic disease is controversial. According to Carson et al. [19], there is an improvement in survival when complete resection of primary tumor or recurrence is performed, especially for those with delayed recurrence (> 12 months from resection of the primary).

The finding that GISTs are characterized by the expression of the transmembrane receptor tyrosine kinase KIT, the product of the c-kit proto-oncogene, and that c-kit is upregulated in this kind of tumors, has recently suggested new alternative treatment approaches to advanced disease. The tyrosine kinase activity of KIT is activated by several different exon mutations in the gene; these mutations result in an activation of the kinase activity with autophosphorylation of the receptor. This in turn leads to a consequent activation of a number of signaling pathways, including mitogen-activated protein kinase and phosphatidyl inositol-3 kinase [20]. The search for inhibitors of these pathways to be used in the treatment of advanced disease started in the 90ies. To date, a number of small molecules have been identified which present a satisfactory inhibitory capacity against the tyrosine kinase activity of KIT.

These compounds were originally developed to target other tyrosine kinases (*e.g.* BCR-ABL). Later studies however showed that their activity was not specific, this becoming helpful with respect to GISTs, because their antitumor efficacy was depending not only on KIT inhibition, but also on the blockade of other kinases that support tumor growth (*e.g.* PDGFR) or its endothelium (VEGF) [21]. Neo-angiogenesis and cell proliferation may be therefore other relevant targets of KIT-inhibitors.

On the other hand, the obtained inhibition of a greater spectrum of molecular functions is linked to an increased frequency of iatrogenic side effects.

Imatinib (STI571) is a new type of tyrosine kinase inhibitor that selectively inhibits various tyrosine kinases. Its low specificity has been used in the treatment of the chronic myelogenous leukemia (CML), where the drug inhibits kinase activity of the BCR-ABL fusion gene product with efficiency, being therefore clinically effective. The drug is administered once-daily by oral administration and is well tolerated. Among the few side effects described is development of mild anemia [22]. The role of this drug in the treatment of GISTs is confirmed by preclinic studies. In essence these preclinical experiences showed rapid inhibition of KIT phosphorylation, with decreased cellular proliferation, and induction of apoptosis after exposure of GIST cells to imatinib mesylate *in vitro* [23].

In vitro study results and the successful treatment of a single patient with metastatic GIST by STI57 have encouraged further studies. A multicenter phase II trial of STI571 in treatment of patients with advanced GIST (unresectable or metastatic GIST) and a phase I study by the European Organization for Research and Treatment of Cancer Soft Tissue and Sarcoma Group was carried out [24]. In this study soft tissues sarcoma were recruited, with the inclusion of GISTs. At the 2001 Annual Meeting of the American Society of Clinical Oncology the preliminary results of the first trial were reported.

In this trial, patients were randomized to receive 400 or 600 mg of STI571 per day. Partial responses after 1- to 3-month therapy were observed in 59% of patients, while disease stabilization was seen in an additional 28% of the cases. The follow-up is quite limited, but only 13% of patients had disease progression. Additionally, clinical improvement was observed in the large majority of patients, and following treatment 89% of the patients with positive fluoro-deoxyglucose positron emission tomography scans had $\geq 50\%$ decreased in the uptake values.

So far, only STI571 has been tested in the treatment of GISTs, but it is possible that KIT TKIs with anti-VEGF receptor activity (*e.g.* SU6668) might have greater activity than ST571 against GIST.

Even though the final results of the multicenter phase II trial are not yet available, the above findings have prompted a phase III Intergroup trial of STI571 for metastatic GIST sponsored by the NCI and, overall, a great, hopefully not exaggerated, enthusiasm for TKIs inhibitors in cancer treatment, depicted also in the media as THE solution for cancer.

Data published in the *New England Journal of Medicine* while this paper was submitted apparently confirm the initial enthusiasm [25].

References

1. Licht JD, Weissmann LB, Antman K. Gastrointestinal sarcomas. *Semin Oncol* 1988; 15: 181-8.
2. Emory T, Sobin L, Lukes L, *et al.* Prognosis of gastrointestinal smooth-muscle (stromal) tumors: dependence on anatomic site. *Am J Surg Pathol* 1999; 23: 82-7.
3. Miettinen M, Sarlomo-Rirala M, Lasota J. Gastrointestinal stromal tumors: recent advances in understanding of their biology. *Hum Pathol* 1999; 30: 1213-20.
4. Myerson RJ, Michalski JM. Gastrointestinal stromal tumors. In: Rustgi AK, ed. *Gastrointestinal cancers: biology, diagnosis, and therapy*. Philadelphia: Lippincott-Raven, 1995: 575-84.
5. Lasota J, Jasinski M, *et al.* Mutations in exon 11 of c-kit occur preferentially in malignant *versus* benign gastrointestinal stromal tumors and do not occur in leiomyomas or leiomyosarcomas. *Am J Pathol* 1999; 154: 53-60.
6. Eilber FC, Rosen G, Forscher C, *et al.* Recurrent gastrointestinal stromal sarcomas. *Surg Oncol* 2000; 9: 71-5.
7. Hasegawa T, *et al.* Gastrointestinal stromal tumor: consistent CD117 immunostaining for diagnosis, and prognosis classification based on tumor size and MIB-1 grade. *Hum Pathol* 2002; 33: 669-76.
8. Kovac D, *et al.* Prognostic factors of gastrointestinal stromal tumors. *Anticancer Res* 2002; 22: 1913-7.
9. Chak A, Canto MI, Rosch T, Dittler HJ. Endosonographic differentiation of benign and malign and stromal cell tumors. *Gastrointest Endosc* 1997; 45: 468-73.
10. Strickland L, Douglas Letson G, Carlos A, Muro-Cacho C. Gastrointestinal stromal tumors. *Cancer Control* 2001: 252-61.
11. Hirata L, Schmitt FC. Gastrointestinal stromal tumors (GIST): morphology and immunoistochemical study of 10 cases. *Arq Gastroenterol* 1991; 28: 55-8.
12. Pfeffel F, Stiglbauer W, Depisch D, *et al.* Coincidence of Crohn's disease and high-risk of gastrointestinal stromal tumors of the terminal ileum. *Digestion* 1999; 60: 363-6.
13. Grant CS, Kim CH, Farruggia G, *et al.* Gastric leiomyosarcoma: prognostic factors and surgical management. *Arch Surg* 1991; 126: 985-90.
14. Ballarini C, Intra M, Ceretti AP, *et al.* Gastrointestinal stromal tumors: a "benign" tumor with hepatic metastasis after 11 years. *Tumori* 1998; 84: 78-81.
15. Yu C, Fletcher C, Newman P, *et al.* A comparison of proliferating cell nuclear antigen (PCNA) immunostaining, nucleolar organizer region stining, and histological grading in gastrointestinal tumors. *J Pathol* 1992; 166: 147-52.
16. Evans HL. Smooth muscle tumors of the gastrointestinal tract: a study of 56 cases for a minimum of 10 years. *Cancer* 1985; 56: 2242-50.
17. Pidhorecky I, Richard T, Cheney W, Kraybill G, Gibbs JF. Gastrointestinal stromal tumors: current diagnosis, biologic behavior, and management. *Ann Surg Oncol* 2000; 7: 705-12.
18. Chen H, Pruitt A, *et al.* Complete hepatic resection of metastases from leiomyosarcoma prolongs survival. *J Gastrointest Surg* 1998; 2: 151-5.
19. Carson W, Karakousis C, Douglas H, *et al.* Results of aggressive treatment of gastric sarcoma. *Ann Surg Oncol* 1994; 1: 244-51.

20. Heinrich MC, Griffith DJ, *et al.* Inhibition of c-kit receptor tyrosine kinase activity by STI571, a selective tyrosine kinase inhibitor. *Blood* 2000; 96: 925-32.
21. Heinrich MC, Blanke CD, Druker BJ, Corless CL. Inhibition of KIT tyrosine kinase activity: a novel molecular approach to the treatment of KIT-positive malignancies. *J Clin Oncol* 2002; 20: 1692-703.
22. Druker BJ, Talpaz M, Resta D, *et al.* Clinical efficacy and safety of an Abl specific TKI as targeted therapy for chronic myelogenous leukemia. *Blood* 1999; 94: 368a.
23. Demetri GD. Targeting c-kit mutations in solid tumors: scientific rationale and novel therapeutic options. *Semin Oncol* 2001; 28 (5 Suppl. 17): 19-26.
24. Joensuu H, Roberts PJ. Effect of the tyrosine kinase inhibitor STI571 in a patient with a metastatic gastrointestinal stromal tumor. *N Engl J Med* 2001; 344: 1052-6.
25. Demetri GD, von Mehren M, Blanke CD, *et al.* Efficacy and safety of imatinib mesylate in advanced gastrointestinal stromal tumors. *N Engl J Med* 2002; 347: 472-80.

Basic mechanisms of liver cancer

Hubert E. Blum, Darius Moradpour

Department of Medicine II, University Hospital Freiburg, Germany

Abstract

Hepatocellular carcinoma (HCC) is one of the most common malignant tumors in some areas of the world with an extremely poor prognosis. The major etiologic risk factors for HCC development include toxins (alcohol, aflatoxin B_1), hepatitis B virus (HBV) and hepatitis C virus (HCV) infection as well as various inherited metabolic disorders, such as alpha-1-antitrypsin deficiency and hemochromatosis.

The molecular mechanisms underlying HCC development are very complex and involve alterations in the structure or expression of several tumor suppressor genes, oncogenes and, possibly, mechanisms leading to a genetic instability due to mismatch repair deficiency or chromosomal instability and aneuploidy due to defective chromosomal segregation. Central to the molecular pathogenesis of HCCs are mutations of various genes and a genetic instability which in most cases results from chronic liver disease and the associated enhanced liver cell regeneration and mitotic activity.

Apart from exploring and refining new HCC treatment strategies, the implementation of existing and the development of novel measures to prevent HCC development are most important. Primary HCC prevention includes among others universal hepatitis B vaccination, antiviral therapy of patients with chronic hepatitis B or C, reduction of food contamination with aflatoxins, elimination of excessive alcohol consumption, etc. Also for some genetic diseases there is the potential for HCC prevention by identifying family members at risk, such as patients with precirrhotic hemochromatosis. Further, secondary prevention of a local HCC recurrence or of new lesions after successful surgical or non-surgical HCC treatment is of paramount importance and is expected to significantly improve disease-free and overall patient survival.

Based on rapid scientific advances, molecular diagnosis, gene therapy and molecular prevention are increasingly becoming part of our patient management and will eventually complement and in part replace existing diagnostic, therapeutic and preventive strategies. Overall, this should result in a reduction of the incidence of HCC, one of the most devastating malignancies worldwide.

Hepatocellular carcinoma (HCC) is one of the most common tumors in the world with an estimated 500,000 to 1,000,000 new cases per year [1]. Although less frequent in the United States and Europe, these tumors have an annual incidence of up to 500 cases per 100,000 population in certain regions of Asia and sub-Saharan Africa. The reasons for this high incidence are chronic infections with the hepatitis B virus (HBV) or the hepatitis C virus (HCV) as well as HBV-HCV coinfections [2-5]. The clinical course of HBV and HCV infection depends in part on the molecular characteristics of the viruses, in part on the patients' HLA haplotype [6, 7], in part on other coexisting risk factors. Well recognized non-viral exogenous agents associated with the pathogenesis of HCC are alcohol and aflatoxins. In the West, alcohol-induced liver injury is a leading cause of liver cirrhosis and the most important HCC risk factor. In Southern China and Africa, dietary ingestion of high levels of aflatoxin B_1 (AFB1) may represent a special environmental hazard, particularly in chronic HBV carriers [8]. Other exogenous factors have also been incriminated and include dietary iron overload [9], long-term use of oral contraceptives and high dose anabolic steroids. The development of liver cirrhosis, particularly in association with genetic diseases, such as alpha-1-antitrypsin deficiency or hemochromatosis, places the individual at a greatly increased risk for the malignant transformation of hepatocytes.

The major clinical risk factor for HCC development is liver cirrhosis since 70-90% of HCCs develop in the setting of a macronodular cirrhosis *(Figure 1)*. The HCC risk in patients with liver cirrhosis depends on the activity, duration and the etiology of the underlying liver disease. In addition, HCCs are more frequent in males than in females and the incidence generally increases with age also in the Western world [10, 11]. In the following we will discuss some targets for the prevention of HCCs, one of the most devastating human malignancies worldwide.

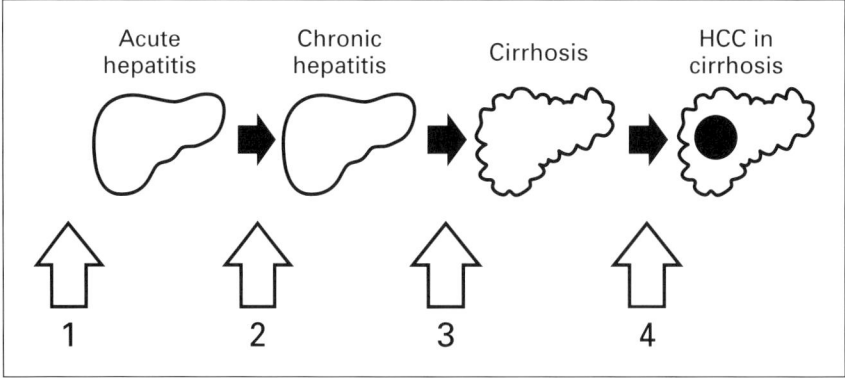

Figure 1. HCC development and primary prevention. **1**: prevention of liver disease, *e.g.* by hygienic measures, prevention of exposure or vaccination against HBV infection, abstinence from alcohol, etc.; **2**: prevention of chronic hepatitis, *e.g.* by treatment of acute hepatitis C, abstinence from alcohol, treatment of hereditary liver diseases, etc.; **3**: prevention of liver cirrhosis, *e.g.* by antiviral treatment of chronic hepatitis B or C, treatment of other chronic liver diseases; **4**: prevention of HCC development in liver cirrhosis, *e.g.* by antiviral treatment, inhibition of fibrosis, etc.

Molecular hepatocarcinogenesis

Central to the concept of molecular carcinogenesis are mutations of oncogenes and tumor suppressor genes as well as genetic instability, including mismatch repair deficiency and impaired chromosomal segregation. In hepatocarcinogenesis, these genetic events occur in the setting of liver cell injury and necrosis associated with an increased rate of hepatocyte regeneration and mitosis. Any exogenous agent, viral or other, that contributes to chronic low grade liver cell damage and mitosis potentially increases the risk of HCC development, rendering liver cell DNA susceptible to additional genetic alterations. Overall, there are a variety of molecular mechanisms by which environmental and viral carcinogens may play a role in HCC development [12, 13].

Oncogenes

Activated cellular oncogenes, particularly those of the *ras* family, have been found in a number of experimental hepatocarcinogenesis models. In human hepatocarcinogenesis, however, no consistent pattern of protooncogene activation has emerged so far for HCC. It is also of interest that no structural or functional changes of a large panel of oncogenes have been found in a transgenic mouse model which is believed to resemble the process of human hepatocarcinogenesis.

Tumor suppressor genes

Restriction fragment length polymorphism studies of paired HCC and non-tumorous liver samples have revealed relatively frequent (> 20% in ≥ 10 informative cases) chromosomal allelic losses (loss of heterozygosity, LOH) in HCC on chromosomes 4, 5q, 8p, 10q, 11p, 13q, 16, 16p and 16q, 17p, and 22q, suggesting that these sites may harbor tumor suppressor genes involved in the pathogenesis of HCC. In general, these genetic alterations appear to occur at later stages of HCC development.

Interestingly, a G to T mutation at the third base position of codon 249 of the p53 gene, leading to a substitution of arginine to serine, was found in a significant number of HCCs in patients from Southern Africa and the Qidong area in China. It was suggested that this "hot spot" mutation was associated with high AFB1 intake in food and may have contributed to the high incidence of HCC in these areas. This finding was supported by *in vitro* studies indicating that the third base of codon 249 of p53 was preferentially targeted to form adducts with AFB1.

DNA mismatch repair genes

In addition to oncogenes and tumor suppressor genes, DNA mismatch repair genes have been identified as a new class of susceptibility genes involved in the pathogenesis of inherited and sporadic human tumors, most notably the hereditary non-polyposis colorectal cancer (HNPCC) [14]. Defective DNA mismatch repair can lead to the accumulation of mutations and microsatellite instability in the cellular genome and thus increase the chance of malignant transformation. The role of DNA mismatch repair defects in HCC development is currently unknown. Recent observations, however, suggest that HBx may interfere with components of the DNA repair machinery [15].

Telomerase activation

The progressive shortening of chromosome ends, or telomeres, accompanies normal cell division and may contribute to cellular aging and serve as a control mechanism against unregulated cellular proliferation. Recently, a remarkable correlation between certain types of cancer and the expression of telomerase, a ribonucleoprotein enzyme preventing the shortening of telomeres, was found. Indeed, expression of telomerase may be a common pathway leading to cancer. In this regard, in a recent study telomerase activity was found in 85% of HCC tissues.

Growth factors

As in most other forms of cancer, the unregulated expression of growth factors and of components of their signalling pathways may play an important role in hepatic oncogenesis. Indeed, overexpression of certain growth factors was found in HCCs, including insulin-like growth factor II, transforming growth factor-alpha and beta, hepatocyte growth factor (HGF), and insulin receptor substrate 1. Surprisingly, HGF has been shown to inhibit the growth of a number of hepatoma cell lines and no neoplasms developed in transgenic mice expressing HGF in the liver under control of the albumin promoter. Moreover, in a study in c-*myc*-HGF double-transgenic mice it was found that coexpression of HGF markedly reduced c-*myc*-induced neoplastic changes The knowledge regarding growth factors in HCC, however, is still incomplete and additional factors are likely to emerge as potentially important candidates involved in hepatocarcinogenesis.

Using oligonucleotide or cDNA microarray expression profiling, suppression substractive hybridization and other methods should allow to further elucidate the genetic events underlying HCC pathogenesis and to identify novel diagnostic markers as well as therapeutic targets [16-18].

Hepatocellular carcinoma natural course

The prognosis of HCC patients is generally very poor. Most studies report a five-year survival rate of less than 5% in symptomatic HCC patients. Furthermore, these tumors have been shown to be quite resistant to radio- or chemotherapy. Investigations of the natural history and clinical course of HCC revealed long-term survival of patients only with small asymptomatic HCCs that could be treated surgically or by non-surgical interventions [19]. Most patients (> 80%) are inoperable at the time of diagnosis. The prognosis of patients with inoperable HCC is very poor, the patient's estrogen receptor status being the strongest prognostic factor for survival [20]. Unfortunately, despite progress in early diagnosis and surgical as well non-surgical treatment strategies, the overall survival of HCC patients has not significantly improved during the last two decades [21]. Preventive strategies, therefore, are of paramount importance and need to be actively explored in order to reduce the incidence of HCCs, one of the most devastating human malignancies worldwide.

Molecular hepatocellular carcinoma therapy

HCC treatment strategies include surgical and non-surgical interventions *(see below)*. Gene therapy for HCC is also being explored *in vitro* as well as in preclinical models and involves three concepts: gene substitution, gene augmentation and DNA vaccination [22, 23].

Gene substitution

One of the most intriguing concepts of gene therapy for cancer is restoration of tumor suppressor function for example by introduction of the wild-type p53 tumor suppressor gene into tumor cells by various gene transfer strategies. Mutations of the p53 tumor suppressor gene are frequently found in HCCs, especially in geographic regions where HBV infection and exposure to AFB1 are risk factors [13]. Loss of wild-type p53 protein function is associated with the malignant phenotype *via* a specific growth or survival advantage for liver cells carrying the p53 mutation and enhances the cellular resistance to a variety of chemotherapeutic drugs [24]. Conversely, introduction of a wild-type p53 gene into HCC cells carrying a mutated p53 gene may result in growth inhibition and restoration of sensitivity to chemotherapeutic drugs. This strategy has been successfully explored *in vitro* by retrovirus mediated transfer of wild-type p53 gene into human HCC cells, resulting in tissue-specific growth inhibition and chemosensitivity to cisplatin [25]. Furthermore, a new and elegant approach uses p53 mutations for selective, adenovirus-mediated lysis of tumor cells. Thus, an adenovirus mutant was engineered that replicates selectively in p53-deficient human tumor cells [26].

Gene augmentation

Gene augmentation is aimed at the local expression of a therapeutic gene product that is physiologically not expressed or expressed at therapeutically insufficient levels. Apart from the expression of cytokines, *e.g.* interleukin-2 (IL-2) or tumor necrosis factor (TNF)-alpha, the therapeutic principle may be a "suicide gene".

Complete regression of a murine HCC has been demonstrated *in vivo* by TNF-alpha [27], by IL-2 [28] as well as by an activatable interferon regulatory factor-1 in mice [29]. Gene transfer was achieved *in vivo* by delivering retroviral [27] or adenoviral vectors [28] systemically, directly into the tumor or into the peritoneal cavity. In principle, gene transfer can also be performed *ex vivo* by transducing tumor infiltrating lymphocytes (TILs) from the patient's HCC with the therapeutic gene, expanding the TILs *in vitro* and giving the *ex vivo* modified TILs back to the patient.

Another strategy to treat HCCs is genetic prodrug activation therapy *via* the introduction of a "suicide gene" into malignant cells followed by the administration of the prodrug.

This concept has been experimentally explored in HCC cells *in vitro* and *in vivo*, e.g. for the HSV-tk gene [30], the gene encoding cytosine deaminase (CD) that converts the prodrug 5-fluorocytosine to 5-fluorouracil which inhibits RNA and DNA synthesis during the S-phase of the cell cycle [31], the gene encoding purine nucleoside phosphorylase that converts purine analogs into freely diffusible toxic metabolites [32, 33] as well as the gene encoding cytochrome p450 4B1 [34]. A significant bystander effect of cell killing caused by suicide gene expression could be demonstrated *in vitro* and *in vivo*, based on cell-cell contact rather than release of cytotoxic substances from the transduced cells. At the same time, the bystander effect may also affect non-malignant dividing cells in the target tissue, potentially limiting the application of this strategy.

DNA vaccination

An elegant and innovative application of gene therapy is the manipulation of the immune system by introduction of expression vectors into muscle cells, resulting in long-lasting cellular and humoral immune responses [35]. DNA-based tumor vaccination against HCC may be possible, for example, by intramuscular introduction of a plasmid expressing HCC-specific antigens or antigens that are highly overexpressed in HCC cells, such as AF-20 antigen, insulin receptor substrate-1, alpha-fetoprotein [36], aspartyl asparaginyl hydroxylase, mutated p53 protein and others. Potential limitations of this strategy include the regulation of the immune response as well as the low level expression of the targeted antigen in non-malignant cells [37], rendering them susceptible to immune mediated elimination as well.

HCC prevention

HCC prevention falls into two categories. Primary prevention that is aimed at the prevention of HCC development in patients with chronic liver diseases of different etiologies and secondary prevention that is aimed at preventing the recurrence and/or the development of new HCC lesions after successful surgical or non-surgical HCC treatment.

Primary hepatocellular carcinoma prevention

Apart from developing and refining novel therapeutic strategies, the implementation of measures for the primary or secondary prevention of HCC development is most important. Primary prevention is aimed at the interference with HCC development at four stages *(Figure 1)*.

Stage 1

Interventions at this step are aimed at the prevention of acquired liver diseases. Apart from avoiding liver toxins, including alcohol and certain drugs, or infections with HBV or HCV by hygienic measures, avoiding parenteral exposure to blood, blood products or contaminated needles, etc., a prime example is vaccination against HBV infection using the commercially available active and passive vaccines. Several HBV vaccines using natural or recombinant hepatitis B surface antigen (HBsAg) from different sources are well introduced in clinical practice and universal vaccination in Taiwan has indeed already resulted in a decline of the incidence of HCCs [38]. In addition, novel HBV vaccination strategies are being explored, including a novel triple HBsAg recombinant vaccine [39], epidermal HBsAg powder immunization [40] as well as oral immunization using HBsAg transgenic plants [41]. Further, DNA vaccination has been shown in animal models to induce antibodies against HBsAg/anti-HBs [42, 43], even after topical application to the skin. For the prevention of HCV infection, however, there is no effective vaccine available to date. While several HCV vaccination concepts are being evaluated, including HCV proteins [44], HCV-like particles [45] as well as intravenous, intrahepatic, intra-epidermal, intramuscular or oral cDNA immunization [46-50], it is not to be expected that a vaccine against HCV infection will become commercially available within the next few years.

Stage 2

Interventions at this step are aimed at the early treatment of acute liver diseases, thereby blocking their transition into chronic hepatitis that carries the risk for developing liver cirrhosis and its sequelae, including HCC. While the principles mentioned above regarding liver toxins also apply here, the early diagnosis and treatment of inherited liver diseases, such as Wilson's disease and hemochromatosis, are of paramount importance. Further, a recent study suggests that early treatment of acute HCV infection prevents its progression to chronic hepatitis C in more than 90% of patients [51].

Stage 3

Interventions at this step are aimed at the prevention of the progression of chronic hepatitis to liver cirrhosis that carries a high risk for HCC development. Apart from avoiding liver toxins, the long-term use of high dose androgens or other anabolic steroids, the treatment of chronic hepatitis is here most important. This includes the treatment of inherited, cholestatic or autoimmune liver diseases as well as the treatment of chronic viral hepatitis B or C. Reduction of iron overload by phlebotomy, for example, has been shown to stop the progression of hemochromatosis to liver cirrhosis and HCC. Treatment of chronic hepatitis B by interferon alpha or nucleoside analogs [52-54] and chronic hepatitis C by interferon alpha and more recently by its combination with the nucleoside analog ribavirin demonstrated biochemical, virological and histopathologial improvement [55-61] and a lower incidence of HCC development [58, 62-64].

Stage 4

Interventions at this step are aimed at interfering with the molecular events leading to HCC development, usually in a cirrhotic liver. These strategies include all treatment modalities detailed above (stage 3) as far as they can be implemented in patients with compensated or decompensated liver cirrhosis [58-61]. In addition, some of the measures to prevent HCC recurrence after successful HCC treatment (secondary prevention, *see below*) should in principle also be useful for HCC prevention at this stage of the liver disease. Further, some concepts of molecular therapy of HCCs *(see above)* should be applicable also for the prevention of HCCs. Without experimental pre-clinical data on these issues it would be premature, however, to discuss their potential clinical impact.

Secondary hepatocellular carcinoma prevention

The prevention of a local recurrence and/or the development of new HCC lesions in patients after successful surgical or non-surgical HCC treatment *(Figure 2)* is of paramount importance and is expected to significantly improve disease-free and overall patient survival.

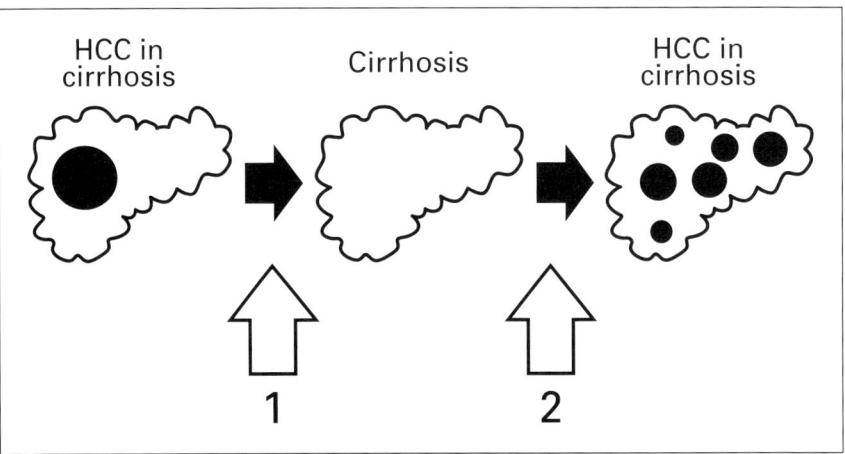

Figure 2. Secondary HCC prevention. **1**: surgical or non-surgical HCC treatment; **2**: prevention local HCC recurrence or new HCC lesions in cirrhotic liver.

Stage 1

HCC treatment strategies include surgical as well as non-surgical interventions. Surgical interventions are resection and in selected cases liver transplantation [65, 66]. Because the majority of patients presents with advanced HCCs at the time of diagnosis or carries a high surgical risk due to comorbidities or advanced age, non-surgical therapeutic interventions are of paramount importance. These include percutaneous ethanol injection (PEI) [67, 68], percutaneous acetic acid injection (PAI) [69], percutaneous thermal ablations, *e.g.* radiofrequencey thermal ablation (RFTA) [70, 71], laser-induced thermal ablation (LiTT) [72] as well as transarterial chemotherapy (TAC), transarterial chemoembolisation (TACE) [67, 73] or transarterial 131-iodine lipiodol therapy. In addition, a number of drugs have been evaluated in clinical trials [74, 75]. While tamoxifen and several chemotherapeutic agents have been shown not to be effective in randomized controlled clinical trials, there are a number of substances that deserve further clinical evaluation, *e.g.* gemcitabine [76, 77], octreotide [78], thymostimulin [79] and pravastatin [80]. Overall, the only potentially curative treatment is surgery, including liver transplantation in selected cases. HCC resection and some non-surgical interventions, especially PEI and RFTA, can prolong disease-free as well as overall survival with survival rates of about 50% at 5 years and in a few cases even result in long-term remission or cure.

Stage 2

After successful HCC resection or non-surgical ablation, HCC recurrence in the remaining, usually cirrhotic liver is the major limitation of the life expectancy of these patients. The probability of recurrence is about 50% within 3 years after successful treatment [65, 81]. Strategies to prevent HCC recurrence are therefore central to the improvement of survival of HCC patients after initial cure. The strategies explored to date include the administration of polyprenoic acid, an acyclic retinoid [82], of interferon alpha [83] and of interferon beta [84]. Further, adoptive immunotherapy [85] and intra-arterial 131-iodine lipiodol treatment [86] have been evaluated in clinical studies. All these interventions have resulted in lower HCC recurrence rates. These findings have to be confirmed, however, in larger randomized controlled studies demonstrating a clear clinical benefit before secondary prevention with one of the strategies mentioned above should enter clinical practice.

Summary and perspectives

HCC is one of the most common malignant tumors in some areas of the world with an extremely poor prognosis. The major etiologic risk factors for HCC development include toxins (alcohol, AFB1), HBV and HCV infection as well as various inherited metabolic disorders, such as alpha-1-antitrypsin deficiency and hemochromatosis.

The molecular pathogenesis of HCC development is very complex and involves alterations in the structure or expression of several tumor suppressor genes, oncogenes and, possibly, mechanisms leading to a genetic instability due to mismatch repair deficiency or chromosomal instability and aneuploidy due to defective chromosomal segregation. Central to the molecular pathogenesis of HCC are mutations of various genes and a genetic instability which in most cases result from chronic liver disease and the associated enhanced liver cell regeneration and mitotic activity.

Gene therapy for HCC falls into three categories: gene replacement, gene augmentation and DNA vaccination. In view of the complexity of the genetic events underlying hepatocarcinogenesis, most studies performed to date have focused on gene augmentation as an experimental therapeutic strategy. Despite exciting prospects of nucleic acid-based HCC therapy, various delivery, targeting and safety aspects need to be addressed before these concepts will enter clinical practice.

Apart from improving HCC therapy, the refinement and implementation of existing as well as the discovery and development of novel strategies aimed at HCC prevention are most important. Primary prevention has been shown to reduce HCC development in some patient groups at risk. For example, hepatitis B vaccination of children in Taiwan has actually resulted in a decline of the HCC incidence. Further, antiviral therapy of patients with chronic hepatitis B or C should contribute to HCC prevention. Public health measures to reduce food contamination with aflatoxins and eliminate excessive alcohol use should also reduce the incidence of chronic liver disease, cirrhosis and thereby HCCs. Apart from primary HCC prevention, interventions aimed at secondary prevention after successful HCC treatment are also a very active area of basic and clinical research. In the future, therefore, preventive measures should have a major impact on reducing the incidence of HCC, one of the most common and devastating malignancies in the world.

References

1. Schafer DF, Sorrell MF. Hepatocellular carcinoma. *Lancet* 1999; 353: 1253-7.
2. Lee WM. Hepatitis B virus infection. *N Engl J Med* 1997; 337: 1733-45.
3. Lauer GM, Walker BD. Hepatitis C virus infection. *N Engl J Med* 2001; 345: 41-52.
4. Di Bisceglie AM. Natural history of hepatitis C: its impact on clinical management. *Hepatology* 2000; 31: 1014-8.
5. Liang TJ, Rehermann B, Seeff LB, Hoofnagle JH. Pathogenesis, natural history, treatment, and prevention of hepatitis C. *Ann Intern Med* 2000; 132: 296-305.
6. Congia M, Clemente MG, Dessi C, et al. HLA class II genes in chronic hepatitis C virus-infection and associated immunological disorders. *Hepatology* 1996; 24: 1338-41.
7. Kuzushita N, Hayashi N, Moribe T, et al. Influence of HLA haplotypes on the clinical courses of individuals infected with hepatitis C virus. *Hepatology* 1998; 27: 240-4.
8. Bailey EA, Iyer RS, Stone MP, Harris TM, Essigmann JM. Mutational properties of the primary aflatoxin B_1-DNA adduct. *Proc Natl Acad Sci USA* 1996; 93: 1535-9.
9. Mandishona E, MacPhail AP, Gordeux VR, et al. Dietary iron overload as a risk factor for hepatocellular carcinoma in black Africans. *Hepatology* 1998; 27: 1563-6.
10. Poynard T, Bedossa P, Opolon P, et al. Natural history of liver fibrosis progression in patients with chronic hepatitis C. *Lancet* 1997; 349: 825-32.
11. El-Serag HB, Mason AC. Rising incidence of hepatocellular carcinoma in the United States. *N Engl J Med* 1999; 340: 745-50.
12. Moradpour D, Wands JR, Blum HE. Molecular biology of hepatitis B and C virus and hepatocellular carcinoma. *Mol Cancer Biol* 1996; 3: 875-904.
13. Ozturk M. Genetic aspects of hepatocellular carcinogenesis. *Semin Liver Dis* 1999; 19: 235-42.
14. Kinzler KW, Vogelstein B. Lessons from hereditary colorectal cancer. *Cell* 1996; 87: 159-70.
15. Becker S, Lee TH, Butel J, Slagle B. Hepatitis B virus X protein interferes with cellular DNA repair. *J Virol* 1998; 72: 266-72.
16. Miyasaka Y, Enomoto N, Nagayama K, et al. Analysis of differentially expressed genes in human hepatocellular carcinoma using suppression subtractive hybridization. *Br J Cancer* 2001; 85: 228-34.
17. Shirota Y, Kaneko S, Honda M, Kawai HF, Kobayashi K. Identification of differentially expressed genes in hepatocellular carcinoma with cDNA microarrays. *Hepatology* 2001; 33: 832-40.
18. Graveel CR, Jatkoe T, Madore SJ, Holt AL, Farnham PJ. Expression profiling and identification of novel genes in hepatocellular carcinomas. *Oncogene* 2001; 20: 2704-12.
19. Yuen MF, Cheng CC, Lauder IJ, Lam SK, Ooi CG, Lai CL. Early detection of hepatocellular carcinoma increases the chance of treatment: Hong Kong experience. *Hepatology* 2000; 31: 330-5.
20. Villa E, Moles A, Ferretti I, et al. Natural history of inoperable hepatocellular carcinoma: estrogen receptors' status in the tumor is the strongest prognostic factor for survival. *Hepatology* 2000; 32: 233-8.
21. El-Serag HB, Mason AC, Key C. Trends in survival of patients with hepatocellular carcinoma between 1977 and 1996 in the United States. *Hepatology* 2001; 33: 62-5.
22. Blum HE, Linhart HG. Gene therapy for hepatocellular carcinoma. *Vir Hepatitis Rev* 1999; 5: 147-57.
23. Blum HE, Moradpour D, Köck J, Tang ZY, von Weizsächer F, Offensperger WB. Gene therapy for hepatocellular carcinoma: concepts and perspectives. In: Fleig W, ed. *Normal and malignant liver cell growth*. Dordrecht, Boston, London, 1999: 232-42.
24. Harris CC. Structure and function of the tumor suppressor gene: clues for rational cancer therapeutic strategies. *J Natl Cancer Inst* 1996; 88: 1442-55.
25. Xu GW, Sun ZT, Forrester K, Wang XW, Coursen J, Harris CC. Tissue-specific growth suppression and chemosensitivity promotion in human hepatocellular carcinoma cells by retroviral-mediated transfer of the wild-type p53 gene. *Hepatology* 1996; 24: 1264-8.
26. Lowe SW. Progress of the smart bomb cancer virus. *Nature Med* 1997; 3: 606-8.

27. Cao G, Kuriyama S, Du P, et al. Complete regression of established murine hepatocellular carcinoma by in vivo tumor necrosis factor alpha gene transfer. *Gastroenterology* 1997; 112: 501-10.
28. Huang H, Chen SH, Kosai K, Finegold MJ, Woo SL. Gene therapy for hepatocellular carcinoma: long-term remission of primary and metastatic tumors in mice by interleukin-2 gene therapy in vivo. *Gene Ther* 1996; 3: 980-7.
29. Kroger A, Ortmann D, Krohne TU, et al. Growth suppression of the hepatocellular carcinoma cell line Hepa1-6 by an activatable interferon regulatory factor-1 in mice. *Cancer Res* 2001; 61: 2609-17.
30. Kanai F, Shiratori Y, Yoshida Y, et al. Gene therapy for alpha-fetoprotein-producing human hepatoma cells by adenovirus-mediated transfer of the herpes simplex virus thymidine kinase gene. *Hepatology* 1996; 23: 1359-68.
31. Kanai F, Lan KH, Shiratori Y, et al. In vivo gene therapy for alpha-fetoprotein-producing hepatocellular carcinoma by adenovirus-mediated transfer of cytosine deaminase gene. *Cancer Res* 1997; 57: 461-5.
32. Mohr L, Shankara S, Yoon SK, et al. Gene therapy of hepatocellular carcinoma in vitro and in vivo in nude mice by adenoviral transfer of the *Escherichia coli* purine nucleoside phosphorylase gene. *Hepatology* 2000; 31: 606-14.
33. Krohne TU, Shankara S, Geissler M, et al. Mechanisms of cell death induced by suicide genes encoding purine nucleoside phosphorylase and thymidine kinase in human hepatocellular carcinoma cells in vitro. *Hepatology* 2001; 34: 511-8.
34. Mohr L, Rainov NG, Mohr UG, Wands JR. Rabbit cytochrome P450 4B1: a novel prodrug activating gene for pharmacogene therapy of hepatocellular carcinoma. *Cancer Gene Ther* 2000; 7: 1008-14.
35. Donnelly JJ, Ulmer JB, Shiver JW, Liu MA. DNA vaccines. *Annu Rev Immunol* 1997; 15: 617-48.
36. Grimm CF, Ortmann D, Mohr L, et al. Mouse alpha-fetoprotein-specific DNA-based immunotherapy of hepatocellular carcinoma leads to tumor regression in mice. *Gastroenterology* 2000; 119: 1104-12.
37. Geissler M, Mohr L, Weth R, et al. Immunotherapy directed against alpha-fetoprotein results in autoimmune liver disease during liver regeneration in mice. *Gastroenterology* 2001; 121: 931-9.
38. Chang MH, Chen CJ, Lai MS, et al. Universal hepatitis B vaccination in Taiwan and the incidence of hepatocellular carcinoma in children. Taiwan Childhood Hepatoma Study Group. *N Engl J Med* 1997; 336: 1855-9.
39. Young MD, Schneider DL, Zuckerman AJ, Du W, Dickson B, Maddrey WC. Adult hepatitis B vaccination using a novel triple antigen recombinant vaccine. *Hepatology* 2001; 34: 372-6.
40. Chen D, Weis KF, Chu Q, et al. Epidermal powder immunization induces both cytotoxic T-lymphocyte and antibody responses to protein antigens of influenza and hepatitis B viruses. *J Virol* 2001; 75: 11630-40.
41. Richter LJ, Thanavala Y, Arntzen CJ, Mason HS. Production of hepatitis B surface antigen in transgenic plants for oral immunization. *Nat Biotechnol* 2000; 18: 1167-71.
42. Davis HL, McClusky MJ, Gerin JL, Purcell H. DNA vaccine for hepatitis B: evidence for immunogenicity in chimpanzees and comparison with other vaccines. *Proc Natl Acad Sci USA* 1996; 93: 7213-8.
43. Prince AM, Whalen R, Brotman B. Successful nucleic acid based immunization of newborn chimpanzees against hepatitis B virus. *Vaccine* 1997; 15: 916-9.
44. Choo QL, Kuo G, Ralston R, et al. Vaccination of chimpanzees against infection by the hepatitis C virus. *Proc Natl Acad Sci USA* 1994; 91: 1294-8.
45. Lechmann M, Murata K, Satoi J, Vergalla J, Baumert TF, Liang TJ. Hepatitis C virus-like particles induce virus-specific humoral and cellular immune responses in mice. *Hepatology* 2001; 34: 417-23.
46. Lee AY, Manning WC, Arian CL, et al. Priming of hepatitis C virus-specific cytotoxic T lymphocytes in mice following portal vein injection of a liver-specific plasmid DNA. *Hepatology* 2000; 31: 1327-33.
47. Weiner AJ, Paliard X, Selby MJ, et al. Intrahepatic genetic inoculation of hepatitis C virus RNA confers cross-protective immunity. *J Virol* 2001; 75: 7142-8.

48. Brinster C, Muguet S, Lone YC, *et al.* Different hepatitis C virus nonstructural protein 3 (Ns3)-DNA-expressing vaccines induce in HLA-A2.1 transgenic mice stable cytotoxic T lymphocytes that target one major epitope. *Hepatology* 2001; 34: 1206-17.
49. Forns X, Payette PJ, Ma X, *et al.* Vaccination of chimpanzees with plasmid DNA encoding the hepatitis C virus (HCV) envelope E2 protein modified the infection after challenge with homologous monoclonal HCV. *Hepatology* 2000; 32: 618-25.
50. Wedemeyer H, Gagneten S, Davis A, Bartenschlager R, Feinstone S, Rehermann B. Oral immunization with HCV-NS3-transformed Salmonella: induction of HCV-specific CTL in a transgenic mouse model. *Gastroenterology* 2001; 121: 1158-66.
51. Jaeckel E, Cornberg M, Wedemeyer H, *et al.* Treatment of acute hepatitis C with interferon alfa-2b. *N Engl J Med* 2001; 345: 1452-7.
52. Malik AH, Lee WM. Chronic hepatitis B virus infection: treatment strategies for the next millennium. *Ann Intern Med* 2001; 132: 723-31.
53. Torresi J, Locarnini S. Antiviral chemotherapy for the treatment of hepatitis B virus infections. *Gastroenterology* 2000; 118: S83-103.
54. Lok AS, Heathcote EJ, Hoofnagle JH. Management of hepatitis B: 2000 – summary of a workshop. *Gastroenterology* 2001; 120: 1828-53.
55. Davis GL. Current therapy for chronic hepatitis C. *Gastroenterology* 2000; 118: S104-14.
56. Manns MP, McHutchison JG, Gordon SC, *et al.* Peginterferon alfa-2b plus ribavirin compared with interferon alfa-2b plus ribavirin for initial treatment of chronic hepatitis C: a randomised trial. *Lancet* 2001; 358: 958-65.
57. Di Bisceglie AM, McHutchison J, Rice CM. New therapeutic strategies for hepatitis C. *Hepatology* 2002; 35: 224-31.
58. Valla DC, Chevallier M, Marcellin P, *et al.* Treatment of hepatitis C virus-related cirrhosis: a randomized, controlled trial of interferon alfa-2b *versus* no treatment. *Hepatology* 1999; 29: 1870-5.
59. Everson GT, Jensen DM, Craig JR, *et al.* Efficacy of interferon treatment for patients with chronic hepatitis C: comparison of response in cirrhotics, fibrotics, or nonfibrotics. *Hepatology* 1999; 30: 271-6.
60. Heathcote EJ, Shiffman ML, Cooksley WG, *et al.* Peginterferon alfa-2a in patients with chronic hepatitis C and cirrhosis. *N Engl J Med* 2000; 343: 1673-80.
61. Poynard T, McHutchison J, Manns M, *et al.* Impact of pegylated interferon alfa-2b and ribavirin on liver fibrosis in patients with chronic hepatitis C. *Gastroenterology* 2002; 122: 1303-13.
62. Yoshida H, Shiratori Y, Moriyama M, *et al.* Interferon therapy reduces the risk for hepatocellular carcinoma: national surveillance program of cirrhotic and noncirrhotic patients with chronic hepatitis C in Japan. Inhibition of Hepatocarcinogenesis by Interferon Therapy Study Group. *Ann Intern Med* 1999; 131: 174-81.
63. Nishiguchi S, Shiomi S, Nakatani S, *et al.* Prevention of hepatocellular carcinoma in patients with chronic active hepatitis C and cirrhosis. *Lancet* 2001; 357: 196-7.
64. Toyoda H, Kumada T, Nakano S, *et al.* Effect of the dose and duration of interferon-alpha therapy on the incidence of hepatocellular carcinoma in noncirrhotic patients with a nonsustained response to interferon for chronic hepatitis C. *Oncology* 2001; 61: 134-42.
65. Llovet JM, Fuster J, Bruix J. Intention-to-treat analysis of surgical treatment for early hepatocellular carcinoma: resection *versus* transplantation. *Hepatology* 1999; 30: 1434-40.
66. Bruix J, Sherman M, Llovet JM, *et al.* Clinical management of hepatocellular carcinoma. Conclusions of the Barcelona-2000 EASL conference. European Association for the Study of the Liver. *J Hepatol* 2001; 35: 421-30.
67. Allgaier HP, Deibert P, Olschewski M, *et al.* Survival benefit of patients with inoperable hepatocellular carcinoma treated by a combination of transarterial chemoembolization and percutaneous ethanol injection – a single-center analysis including 132 patients. *Int J Cancer* 1998; 79: 601-5.

68. Yamamoto J, Okada S, Shimada K, *et al.* Treatment strategy for small hepatocellular carcinoma: comparison of long-term results after percutaneous ethanol injection therapy and surgical resection. *Hepatology* 2001; 34: 707-13.
69. Ohnishi K, Yoshioka H, Ito S, Fujiwara K. Prospective randomized controlled trial comparing percutaneous acetic acid injection and percutaneous ethanol injection for small hepatocellular carcinoma. *Hepatology* 1998; 27: 67-72.
70. Grasso A, Watkinson AF, Tibballs JM, Burroughs AK. Radiofrequency ablation in the treatment of hepatocellular carcinoma – a clinical viewpoint. *J Hepatol* 2000; 33: 667-72.
71. Morimoto M, Sugimori K, Shirato K, *et al.* Treatment of hepatocellular carcinoma with radiofrequency ablation: radiologic-histologic correlation during follow-up periods. *Hepatology* 2002; 35: 1467-75.
72. Giorgio A, Tarantino L, de Stefano G, *et al.* Interstitial laser photocoagulation under ultrasound guidance of liver tumors: results in 104 treated patients. *Eur J Ultrasound* 2000; 11: 181-8.
73. Bruix J, Llovet JM, Castells A, *et al.* Transarterial embolization *versus* symptomatic treatment in patients with advanced hepatocellular carcinoma: results of a randomized, controlled trial in a single institution. *Hepatology* 1998; 27: 1578-83.
74. Simonetti RG, Liberati A, Angiolini C, Pagliaro L. Treatment of hepatocellular carcinoma: a systematic review of randomized controlled trials. *Ann Oncol* 1997; 8: 117-36.
75. Mathurin P, Rixe O, Carbonell N, *et al.* Review article: Overview of medical treatments in unresectable hepatocellular carcinoma – an impossible meta-analysis? *Aliment Pharmacol Ther* 1998; 12: 111-26.
76. Yang TS, Lin YC, Chen JS, Wang HM, Wang CH. Phase II study of gemcitabine in patients with advanced hepatocellular carcinoma. *Cancer* 2000; 89: 750-6.
77. Kubicka S, Rudolph KL, Tietze MK, Lorenz M, Manns M. Phase II study of systemic gemcitabine chemotherapy for advanced unresectable hepatobiliary carcinomas. *Hepatogastroenterology* 2001; 48: 783-9.
78. Kouroumalis E, Skordilis P, Thermos K, Vasilaki A, Moschandrea J, Manousos ON. Treatment of hepatocellular carcinoma with octreotide: a randomised controlled study. *Gut* 1998; 42: 442-7.
79. Palmieri G, Biondi E, Morabito A, Rea A, Gravina A, R. BA. Thymostimulin treatment of hepatocellular carcinoma on liver cirrhosis. *Int J Oncol* 1996; 8: 827-32.
80. Kawata S, Yamasaki E, Nagase T, *et al.* Effect of pravastatin on survival in patients with advanced hepatocellular carcinoma. A randomized controlled trial. *Br J Cancer* 2001; 84: 886-91.
81. Koike Y, Shiratori Y, Sato S, *et al.* Risk factors for recurring hepatocellular carcinoma differ according to infected hepatitis virus – an analysis of 236 consecutive patients with a single lesion. *Hepatology* 2000; 32: 1216-23.
82. Muto Y, Moriwaki H, Ninomiya M, *et al.* Prevention of second primary tumors by an acyclic retinoid, polyprenoic acid, in patients with hepatocellular carcinoma. Hepatoma Prevention Study Group. *N Engl J Med* 1996; 334: 1561-7.
83. Kubo S, Nishiguchi S, Hirohashi K, *et al.* Effects of long-term postoperative interferon-alpha therapy on intrahepatic recurrence after resection of hepatitis C virus-related hepatocellular carcinoma. A randomized, controlled trial. *Ann Intern Med* 2001; 134: 963-7.
84. Ikeda K, Arase Y, Saitoh S, *et al.* Interferon beta prevents recurrence of hepatocellular carcinoma after complete resection or ablation of the primary tumor. A prospective randomized study of hepatitis C virus-related liver cancer. *Hepatology* 2000; 32: 228-32.
85. Takayama T, Sekine T, Makuuchi M, *et al.* Adoptive immunotherapy to lower postsurgical recurrence rates of hepatocellular carcinoma: a randomised trial. *Lancet* 2000; 356: 802-7.
86. Lau WY, Leung TW, Ho SK, *et al.* Adjuvant intra-arterial iodine-131-labelled lipiodol for resectable hepatocellular carcinoma: a prospective randomised trial. *Lancet* 1999; 353: 797-801.

Liver cancer.
Multimodality approaches to treatment

P. Schemmer, A. Mehrabi, P. Büchler, A.A. Tempia-Caliera,
H. Friess, M.W. Büchler

Department of General Surgery, University of Heidelberg, Heidelberg, Germany

Abstract

The only potential cure of liver malignancy is limited to surgical interventions, i.e. *liver resection or transplantation. Unfortunately, tumors often are discovered in advanced stages in which surgical therapy alone is not enough. Today, the management of hepatic malignancy is one of the most controversial areas in medicine. This continuously evolving field includes a multimodal approach of treatment which requires cooperation of medical oncologists, hepatobiliary surgeons, radiotherapists, interventional radiologists and in few cases transplant surgeons. Further, the most recent developments of neoadjuvant cancer therapy, cryosurgery, thermoablative techniques and immunological manipulation of tumor cells and others have added to the complexity in the field of approaches to treatment of liver malignancy. However, the use of multimodal approaches described here should be limited to centers with an experienced team. First in line is a surgeon experienced with difficult hepatectomies. Mortality following major hepatectomy is below 5% in centers of reference [1]. This chapter reviews the current literature with the focus on effective multimodal treatment options of both the two most common primary malignant liver tumors (hepatocellular carcinoma (HCC), cholangiocarcinoma (CCC)) and metastases to the liver predominantly derived from colorectal cancer. For later hepatic malignancy about 50% of patients underwent liver resection at our institution during the last 7 months compared with about 8% and 5% patients with HCC or CCC, respectively. These numbers roughly display the actual prevalence of hepatic malignancy in patients.*

Major hepatic resection

The development of hepatobiliary surgery culminates in the rise and increased safety of hepatic resections. Complications after liver resection comprise blood loss, liver failure, hematoma, infections, and bile leakage. Advances in the methods of both vascular control and surgically based resections limit morbidity and mortality to postoperative complications unrelated to blood loss [2]. This is especially important for patients undergoing liver resection for malignancy. The recurrence-free survival of patients with hepatocellular carcinoma (HCC) without intrahepatic metastases, who require blood transfusion after potential curative resection, is significantly shorter compared to transfusion free patients [3]. Since surgical technique is a major factor to prevent complications, various techniques have been developed for safe and tissue preserving dissection of the liver parenchyma. Blunt dissection using the finger fracture technique, dissectors using ultrasound, jet water stream, laser or specially prepared suction devices are developed. The introduction of new surgical instruments have permitted large, non-anatomical wedge resections in a relatively bloodless field without hepatic inflow occlusion and ischemia/reperfusion of liver tissue being associated with postoperative liver dysfunction. With reduction of operative mortality to below 5% in patients that undergo extended hepatic resection [1, 4, 5], elective liver surgery has gained acceptance as the primary mode of therapy for many primary and metastatic tumors of the liver. Most data relate to colorectal metastases. In these cases survival time ranges from 4.5 to 15 months [6] which can be prolonged by liver resection with curative intent to about 37 months [7, 8]. Five-year survival following primary and repeat liver resections for colorectal metastases is consistently reported as 25-33% *(Table I)* and has not been improved significantly by adjuvant chemotherapy [7, 9]. Patients with potentially resectable but untreated HCC have been reported to have a median survival time of less than six months [10] and no 5-year survival has yet been reported [11]. However, most recent data reveal that surgical therapy prolongs the median survival to 42 months and 5-year survival can be achieved in 31% to 51% of cases [12, 13] *(Table I)*.

Table I. 5-year survival after liver resection in single center series since 1990 with a) more than 200 patients with liver metastases or HCC; b) in series since 2000 with more than 100 patients with CCC

Author	Reference	Year	No. of patients	Patient survival (%)			Tumor
				1 year	3 years	5 years	
a)							
Scheele et al.	[40]	1991	207	–	–	33	MCC[1]
Rosen et al.	[41]	1992	280	–	–	25	MCC
Gayowski et al.	[42]	1994	301	–	–	32	MCC
Scheele et al.	[43]	1995	434	–	–	33	MCC
Nordlinger et al.	[44]	1996	1,568	–	–	28	MCC
Jamison et al.	[45]	1997	280	–	–	27	MCC
Jaeck et al.	[7]	1997	1,818	–	–	26	MCC
Bakalakos et al.	[46]	1998	301	–	–	29	MCC
Fong et al.	[47]	1999	1,001	–	–	31	MCC
Iwatsuki et al.	[48]	1999	305	–	–	32	MCC
Yamanaka et al.	[33]	1990	295	76	44	31	HCC[2]
Nagasue et al.	[34]	1993	229	80	51	26	HCC
Lai et al.	[36]	1995	343	60	33	24	HCC
Takenaka et al.	[35]	1996	280	88	70	50	HCC
Hanazaki et al.	[37]	2000	386	–	–	34	HCC
Kanematsu et al.	[13]	2002	303	84	67	51	HCC
b)							
Lillemoe et al.	[38]	2000	109	68	30	17.5	CCC[3]
Lee et al.	[39]	2000	111	97.1	55.3	24	CCC

[1] MCC: metastatic colorectal cancer; [2] HCC: hepatocellular carcinoma; [3] CCC: cholangiocellular carcinoma.

Surgical approach

A large variety of incisions are used, including subcostal incision with possible extension as a median sternotomy or right thoracotomy and a midline or paramedian incision in liver surgery. Based on the lobar and segmental liver anatomy determined by the portal and the major hepatic veins, four types of major resection have been employed: right hepatic lobectomy *(Figure 1a)*, left hepatic lobectomy *(Figure 1a)*, right trisegmentectomy (resection of the right lobe with the medial segment of the left lobe) *(Figure 1e)*, and left lateral segmentectomy *(Figure 1b)*. Since most of the malignant tumors respect the intrahepatic boundaries, this approach for liver resection for malignant tumors offers superior tumor clearance and probably better long-term outcome. With improved resection techniques, more categories of liver resection have been applied [14]. Occasionally the left trisegmentectomy (resection of the left lobe plus the anterior segment of the right lobe) *(Figure 1e)* and left medial segmentectomy (left middle lobectomy) *(Figure 1b)* are performed in most centers. While lobectomy and trisegmentectomy require hilar dissection, left lateral segmentectomy does not. Segment-orientated resections are defined by additional use of the transverse boundaries of the cranially and caudally directed third-order ramification of the portal trunks. Despite the advantage of anatomical resections, there are rational indications for non-anatomical procedures such as removal of small benign tumors, excision of HCC in liver cirrhosis, re-resection following major hepatectomy, and excision biopsy in a non-resectable situation. In general, routine use of intraoperative ultrasound, maintenance of a low central venous pressure during dissection of parenchyma, intermittent hilar clamping, and ischemic as well as other preconditioning of liver all contribute to an oncologically effective and safe surgical procedure. Moreover, augmentation of the liver remnant by preoperative portal vein embolization and multicenter trials on multidisciplinary strategies may help to enhance resectability and to further improve both safety and long-term outcome.

Right hemihepatectomy

In patients undergoing right hemihepatectomy, the anterior approach can be used as an alternative to the conventional procedure in which the right liver lobe is completely mobilized [15]. The vena cava is exposed from the lateral aspect, and the veins entering it from the right half of the liver are divided outside the organ prior to dividing the liver parenchyma. Especially, in cases of large or capsule-brooding tumors of the right liver lobe, exposure of the retrohepatic vena cava from the anterior aspect facilitates work on dissection of the hepatic veins [16]. The right liver lobe needs not to be moved and perfusion of the remnant liver and the venous return *via* the vena cava remains unimpaired during surgery. Thus, the no-touch technique is applicable with the anterior approach and tumor manipulation is minimal with minimized risk of iatrogenic tumor perforation or hematogenous dissemination of malignant cells during surgery [17]. Using the anterior approach, a radical en bloc resection is facilitated; however, these benefits are associated with an increased risk of bleeding from hepatic veins during dissection of the parenchyma. Since, the right lobe of the liver is not mobilized, such bleeding is frequently difficult to deal with [15, 18].

	Anatomical term	Couinaud´segments referred to	Term for surgical resection
a	Right hemiliver or right liver	Segment V – VIII (± Sg1)	Right hepatectomy or right hemihepatectomy (stipulate ± segment)
	Left hemiliver or left liver	Segment II – IV (± Sg1)	Left hepatectomy or left hemihepatectomy (stipulate ± segment)
b	Right anterior section	Segment V, VIII	Add (-ectomy) to any of the anatomical terms as in right anterior sectionectomy
	Right posterior section	Segment VI, VII	Right posterior sectionectomy
	Left medial section	Segment IV	Left medial sectionectomy or resection segment IV (also see Third order) or segmentectomy IV (also see Third order)
	Left lateral section	Segment II, III	Left lateral sectionectomy or bisegmentectomy II, III (also see Third order)
c	Segments I – X	Any one of segment I to IX	Segmentectomy (e.g. segmentectomy VI)
	Two continuous segments	Any two of sg I to sg IX in continuity	Bisegmentectomy (e.g. bisegmentectomy V, VI)

	Anatomical term	Couinaud'segments referred to	Term for surgical resection	Diagram (pertinent area is dark)
d	Right anterior sector or right paramedian sector	Segment V, VIII	Add (-ectomy) to any of the anatomical terms as in right anterior sectorectomy or right paramedian sectorectomy	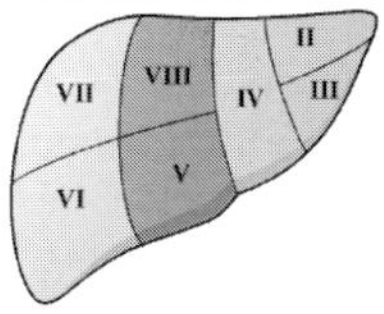
	Right posterior sector or right lateral sector	Segment VI, VII	Right posterior sectorectomy or right lateral sectorectomy	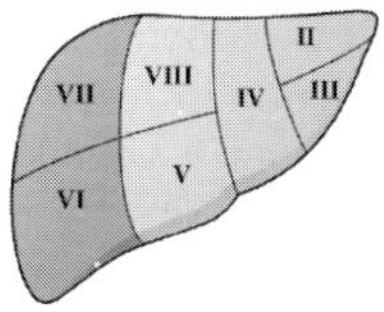
	Left medial sector or left paramedian sector	Segment III, IV	Left medial sectorectomy or left paramedian sectorectomy or bisegmentectomy III, IV	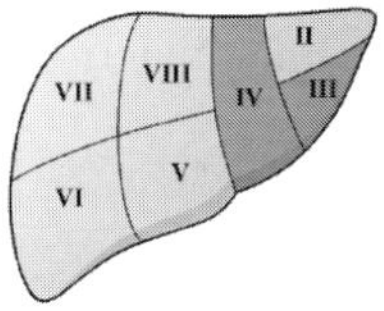
	Left lateral sector or left posterior sector	Segment II	Left lateral sectorectomy or left posterior sectorectomy or segmentectomy II	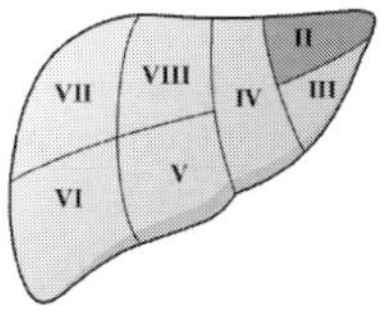
e		Segment IV – VIII (+/-Sgl)	Right trisectionectomy (preferred term) or extended right hepatectomy or extended right hemihepatectomy (stipulate ± segment)	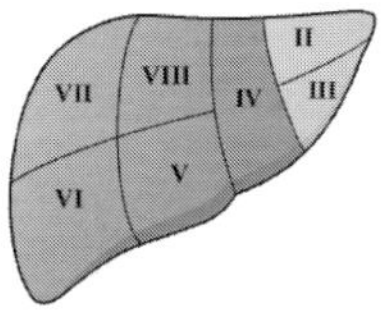
		Segment II, III, IV, V, VIII (± Sgl)	Left trisectionectomy (preferred term) or extended left hepatectomy or extended left hemihepatectomy (stipulate ± segment)	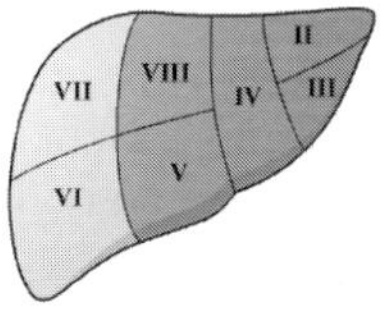

Figure 1. The Brisbane 2000 terminology of hepatic anatomy and resection. a: first-order division: the so-called midplane of the liver is a plane which intersects the fossa of the gallbladder and the fossa for the inferior vena cava (IVC), which is the dividing line of the first order division, separating the two liver lobes; b: second-order division: based on hepatic artery and bile ducts; c: third-order division: the dividing line of the segments are planes called intersegmental planes. Here segments 1 and 9 are not displayed. According to the Brisbane 2000 terminology, it is allowed to name any resection by its removed third-order segments; d: alternative second-order division based on portal vein (PV); e: alternative second-order division based on PV: the dividing line of second-order division based on PV are called right and left intersectional planes. There are no surface markings; f: further liver resections based on liver sections: the dividing line of the sections are planes called right and left intersectional planes. The left intersectional plane goes through the umbilical fissure and the attachment of the falciform ligament. On the right intersectional plane is no surface marking.

Hilar resection

Limited rates of both resectability (80%) and radicallity are reported with low mortality (< 5%) after hilar resection and hemihepatectomy as surgical therapy for hilar cholangiocarcinoma [19-23]. To increase the number of resectable patients as well as their long-term survival, the general principles of surgical oncology have to be applied [22]. Due to the architecture of the hepatic hilum and side-specific variations within the biliary tree, right trisegmentectomy *(Figure 1e)* and principal portal vein resection have the potential to comply with basic rules of surgical oncology, such as wide tumor-free resection margins and no-touch resection technique. After preoperative portal embolization, extended liver resection or formally curative right trisegmentectomy *(Figure 1e)* and portal vein resection excellent 5-year survival rates can be achieved even in cases of advanced tumor stages [20]. Resection of the entire biliary tract without dissection of the tumor is possible by combining total hepatectomy, partial pancreatoduodenectomy and liver transplantation. However, even with this procedure, metastases implantation and tumor recurrence are inevitable due to post-transplant immunosuppression [24].

Laparoscopic liver resection

The potential advantages of laparoscopic liver resections can be summarized with reduced postoperative pain and hospital stay, decreased peritoneal adhesions, cosmetic advantage, less postoperative immune dysfunction and earlier access to adjuvant treatment for malignant disease by fast recovery. These supposed advantages apply especially to patients who undergo liver resection for malignant lesions, including metastatic disease, mostly of colorectal origin, and HCC. However, there is a debate about the specific risks of tumor seeding during laparoscopic surgery. While early attempts at laparoscopic resection of cancer were associated with high numbers of abdominal metastases, especially at port sites, but also in the peritoneal cavity [25], most recent prospective studies ensuring proper oncological surgery with no-touch technique, specimen bag, and abdominal wall protection do not confirm this trend [26]. Thus, mechanisms for tumor seeding include most likely direct contamination by technical errors. Therefore, the lesion to be resected should be reasonably small, because large tumors are more difficult to mobilize, have more dangerous vascular connections, and have a higher risk of bleeding [27]. The potential risk of gas embolism led some surgeons to use gasless suspension laparoscopy [28]. In cases CO_2 is used, which is highly soluble, gas embolism is rare [29]. Portal hypertension and ascites are major risk factors for the development of postoperative decompensation after open resection. The laparoscopic approach may be beneficial for these patients since the abdominal wall is preserved and interruption of collateral veins hereby prevented. Further, the abdominal viscera are not exposed with laparoscopic procedures and both less need for fluid resuscitation and improved reabsorption of ascites is given [27]. To date, the technical complexity of liver surgery, the risk of life-threatening bleeding, and the fear of gas embolism have withheld many from embarking on laparoscopic liver surgery; however, with greater experience in both laparoscopy and liver surgery, laparoscopic liver resection is now feasible and safe in selected patients with left sided and right-peripheral lesions requiring limited resection [27]. Randomized studies are still pending, which show an advantage of laparoscopic liver resection compared with open liver surgery.

Ex situ liver resection

In most cases of liver tumors, resection can be performed with standard techniques. To better control intraoperative blood flow to the liver, partial or total vascular occlusion can be applied when needed. The time of tolerable warm ischemia has yet not been well defined; however, even more than 60 minutes of warm ischemia of liver has been reported to be safe. In a few patients liver protection by hypothermic perfusion is advantageous after extended vascular resection and reconstruction. This can be performed by *in situ* perfusion, *ante situm* resection and *ex situ* resection [30-32]. Further, major reconstruction of hepatic vessels should be performed under *in situ* hypothermic protection using a veno-venous bypass [31]. Both the *in situ* and *ante situm* resection can be used in patients with tumors involving the hepatic venous confluence and/or the retrohepatic vena cava [30]. Only in very few oncological cases there is an indication for *ex situ* liver resection with subsequent autotransplantation of the remnant liver [30].

Outcome after liver resection for liver malignancy

Hepatobiliary surgery, *i.e.* liver resection, is the treatment of choice for liver malignancy. Several studies have documented the benefit of liver resection for patients who underwent resection for HCC [13, 33-37], CCC [38, 39] and liver metastases [7, 40-48] *(Table I)*.

Liver transplantation

Although surgical resection for HCC and CCC is the treatment of choice affording the best outcome, many patients have tumors that are unresectable. For these patients, orthotopic liver transplantation (OLT) theoretically provides the opportunity for wide resection margins. In Europe, OLT is performed for malignant liver tumors in about 12% of recipients [49]; however, the allocation of limited donor organs to this population of patients has been extremely controversial especially since the use of living donors and domino liver transplantation might not be enough to successfully expand the donor pool. In the literature, several centers reported the use of OLT for patients with HCC or CCC with limited results because of high recurrence rates [50-59]; however, it is generally accepted that OLT for HCC can be recommended for a small single tumor with < 5 cm in size, in cases of multiple lesions (≤ 3 nodules) each ≤ 3 cm in diameter and/or unresectable tumors in patients with cirrhosis and without evidence of vascular invasion or extra-hepatic tumor growth [60, 61]. Five-year actuarial survival rates with OLT vary between 18% and 78%, depending on the stage of disease and use of additional chemotherapy *(Table II)*. Klintmalm analyzed 422 patients collected by the International Registry of Hepatic Tumors in Liver Transplantation. Interestingly, patients in whom HCC was found incidentally at the time of surgery had the same prognosis as patients transplanted for tumors [62]. In early series of transplantation for CCC, the vast majority of patients did not survive for more than 3 years; however, recent single-center data reveal that 5-year survival can be achieved in 10% to 36% of cases *(Table II)*. Although these outcomes represent significant improvements over palliative cancer therapies, they are clearly inferior to outcomes after OLT for non-malignant indications.

Table II. 5-year survival after liver transplantation for HCC or CCC in series since 1990 with more than 20 patients in total

Author	Reference	Year	No. of patients	Patient survival (%)			Tumor
				1 year	3 years	5 years	
Penn et al.	[50]	1991	165	30		18	HCC[1]
Colella et al.	[52]	1997	71	96	81	81	HCC
Figueras et al.	[53]	2000	85	84	76	60	HCC
Iwatsuki et al.	[51]	2000	220	68	46	37	HCC
Tamura et al.	[54]	2001	53	87	81	78	HCC
O'Grady et al.	[56]	1987	13	38	10	10	CCC[2] (IH[a])
			13	30	10	10	CCC (EH[b])
Pichlmayr et al.	[57]	1996	25	60	21.4	17.1	CCC (EH)
Casavilla et al.	[58]	1997	20	70	29	18	CCC (IH)
Iwatsuki et al.	[59]	1998	27	59.3	36.2	36.2	CCC (EH)

[1] HCC: hepatocellular carcinoma; [2] CCC: cholangiocellular carcinoma; [a] IH: intrahepatic; [b] EH: extrahepatic.

Neoadjuvant/adjuvant/palliative therapy

In most series, only a small number of liver tumors are resectable at the time of diagnosis for various reasons and options for further improvement of prognosis by purely technical means in surgery appear limited. Instead, future strategies aim to increase the number of patients amenable for potentially curative liver resection. Indeed, to date, advances in imaging technology can identify early resectable lesions. In addition prognosis can be improved by the combination of surgical resection with local ablative measures, neoadjuvant treatment, and selective portal embolization to increase the volume of remnant liver. Recent advances in interdisciplinary measures, which can be combined for treatment of liver tumors, improved the overall prognosis of patients with primary or secondary hepatic malignancy.

Preoperative portal embolization to induce hypertrophy of the liver

About 80 years ago Rous and Larimore observed that ligation of portal venous branches leads to an atrophy of dependent liver parenchyma and hypertrophy of the contralateral liver lobe based on proliferation of both hepatocytes and endothelial cells. Preoperative portal embolization (PVE) has now been established to a world wide used technology to induce hypertrophy of the anticipated liver remnant [63, 64]. In non-cirrhotic livers the volume of proliferated tissue is between 12 cm^3 to 21 cm^3 per day within the first two weeks after PVE. In contrast, the rate of proliferation in cirrhotic liver is only about 9 cm^3 per day. The increment of the anticipated remnant liver volume is about 12% (range: 7% to 27%) of total liver volume and the resection rate after PVE can be increased from 58% to 100% [65-67]. Preoperative PVE is effective to be used in cases of central located liver tumors that can only be resected together with large volumes of intact liver tissue, *i.e.* in cases of hilar or diffuse cholangiocarcinoma, small carcinoma with infiltration of the right portal venous branch or small multifocal malignant lesions in the right liver lobule. PVE is not needed if the remnant liver volume is expected to exceed approximately 30-40%

of total liver volume. Complications of PVE are rare; however, transient hemobilia, ileus of small bowel and reduced arterial blood flow to the liver are reported in up to 10% of all cases.

Therefore, preoperative PVE for major hepatic resection is a safe procedure, which neither improves nor worsens long-term prognosis but is very effective in increasing the safety of surgery or expanding resectability in patients that, otherwise, are considered unresectable. However, indications and beneficial effects of PVE are still under discussion [63, 64, 67].

Chemotherapy

In some of these patients neoadjuvant chemotherapy can downstage the tumor and makes subsequent curative resection applicable. Protocols with fluorouracil (5-FU) alone are useless in the neoadjuvant setting, since response rates of about 10-20% in patients with colorectal liver metastases are disappointing [68]. Regional chemotherapy into the hepatic artery results in significantly higher response rates (about 40-50%) with subsequent success in secondary curative liver resection of initially unresectable colorectal liver metastases; however, regional chemotherapy is invasive and therefore not a standard procedure for every patient with colorectal liver metastases [69]. Recently new promising treatment options have become available for colorectal cancer. Neoadjuvant chemotherapy with irinotecan + 5-FU + folinic acid (FA) or oxaliplatin + 5-FU + FA results in response rates of 50% and can be considered a new standard first-line therapy for patients with metastatic colorectal cancer. Most recently, beneficial effects of neoadjuvant chronomodulated chemotherapy with oxaliplatin + 5-FU + FA have been achieved for patients with unresectable colorectal liver metastases [70, 71]. Fifty-three patients were converted to a resectable stage with 3- and 5-year survival rates of 54% and 40% respectively [70]. In contrast, HCC in general is one of the most resistant tumors to chemotherapy. No single drug or drug combination has shown a response rate more than 20% [72]. Thus systemic chemotherapy is only indicated for HCC in patients in whom the 3 standard treatments – resection-transplantation, percutaneous intralesional ethanol injection (PEI), transcatheter arterial chemoembolization (TACE) – are contraindicated [72]. No benefit has been reported with the use of chemotherapy alone in CCC; however, Verbeek *et al.* reported that adjuvant treatment in patients after non-curative resection improved median survival to 27 months compared with 8 months [1].

Cryotherapy/cryosurgery

Currently performed *via* laparotomy, laparoscopy or percutaneous cryotherapy/cryosurgery is an effective and precise technique for inducing tumor necrosis *via* thermal mechanisms. Reports of two-year survival after cryotherapy for treatment of liver metastases have ranged from 12% to 72% with a local recurrence rate of about 44% [73]. To date there are more than 1,000 patients treated with cryotherapy with a perioperative mortality of 0.9% to 7% [73, 74]. HCCs of 5 cm or less in diameter show a remarkable response in a retrospective analysis of 113 cases, with 5-year and 10-year survival rates of 49% and 17%, respectively, compared with 22% and 8% in the whole series including larger tumors [72].

Percutaneous local ethanol injection (PEI)

It results in an inhomogeneous distribution in liver metastases with unreliable control rates. Relative contraindications to this technique include lesions > 5 cm in size, subcapsular lesions and proximity to bile vessels [1]. Almost all tumors smaller than 2 cm in diameter can be completely ablated in a single session. Long-term survival after ethanol injection for HCC is reported with rates of 83% and 34% after 1 year and 4 years, respectively [75] *(Table III)*. In more than 50% of cases of liver metastasis less than 4 cm in size, complete necrosis can be obtained [76]. In small HCCs the technique has been shown to have equivalent survival to surgery with about 80% for resection and about 70% for PEI [77] *(Table III)*. Serious complications are rare. The most common problems are pain and a feeling of intoxication immediately after the procedure. Fever and pain may occur some days later associated with necrosis of the tumor.

Table III. 5-year survival after percutaneous local ethanol injection for HCC in series since 1990 with ≥ 100 patients

Author	Reference	Year	No. of patients	Patient survival (%)			Tumor
				1 year	3 years	5 years	
Shiina et al.	[92]	1993	146	79	46	38	HCC[1]
Lencioni et al.	[93]	1995	105	96	68	32	HCC
Livraghi et al.	[94]	1995	470	96	63	39	HCC

Tumor size ranged from ≤ 2 cm to 6.5 cm. [1] HCC : hepatocellular carcinoma.

Arterial infusion of chemotherapy

Isolated hepatic perfusion (IHP) is a specialized surgical technique in which the inflow and outflow of the liver are isolated, connected to an extracorporal bypass circuit, and perfused with an anticancer agent in the setting of hyperthermia. In recent studies, after achieving the adequate tissue hyperthermia of 38.5°C to 40°C, chemotherapy, *i.e.* melphalan + cisplatin, mitomycin C, melphalan + TNF, and melphalan + floxuridine + leucovorin, was administered and perfused for about 60 minutes in patients with liver metastases [78, 79]. There was significant treatment mortality in some studies up to 33% with melphalan + TNF; however, in general there was a response rate in up to 77% of cases dependent on the administered chemotherapeutic regimen [78]. For obtaining near total vascular isolation of the liver percutaneous IHP can be used. Several clinical trials and phase I studies used doxorubicin for patients with unresectable HCC and liver metastases from colorectal cancer [78]. Although a large percentage of patients initially respond to IHP-therapy, most have recrudescent disease within 1 year [79].

Transarterial chemoembolization (TACE)

This combines intra-arterial infusion of an anti-cancer agent with particle embolization, inducing both selective ischemic and targeted chemotherapeutic effects. Many embolic agents, *i.e.* gelatine, sponge, starch, polyvinyl ethanol, collagen, cyanoacrylate, lipidol and others, have been used in association with adriamycin, cisplatin, mitomycin, epirubicin or styrene-maleic-acid-neocarzinostatin [75, 80]. Complications include nausea, fever, abdominal pain, abscess formation, jaundice and encephalopathy. After TACE with gelatine sponge particles and doxorubicin or mitomycin for HCC about 75% of patients showed a response with an overall median survival of only 13 months [72]. In other studies, survival after 1/2 years was 62%/26% without cirrhosis and 18%/9% with cirrhosis, respectively [72] *(Table IV)*. Further, median survival time of patients with colorectal metastases in the liver after TACE, especially with 5-FU + leucovorin, has been reported to be from 8 to 14 months, which is in the same range as historical controls treated with systemic chemotherapy [80].

Table IV. 2-year survival after transarterial chemoembolization for HCC in series since 1990 with ≥ 50 patients

Author	Reference	Year	No. of patients	Patient survival (%) 1 year	Patient survival (%) 2 years	Tumor
Bronowicki et al.*	[88]	1994	127	64	38	HCC
Stefanini et al.*	[89]	1995	69	73	44	HCC
Groupe d'Étude/ Traitement du HCC	[90]	1995	50	62	38	HCC
Pelletier et al.	[91]	1998	73	53	25	HCC

* Significant compared with conservative treatment (p < 0.001).

Thermal ablation

Localized hyperthermia can be achieved by radiofrequency, microwave or laser therapy. To date, there is insufficient data for comparison of the various techniques; however, they are highly effective debulking techniques.

In **radiofrequency ablation** (RFA), alternating electrical current generated in the liver tissue from a needle electrode induces friction heat that leads to coagulative necrosis, which can be assessed immediately using CT, MRI or doppler ultrasound [72, 75]. RFA has been recommended for cirrhotic patients with liver tumors less than 5 cm in diameter *(Table V)*. There is evidence that RFA provides local short-term control of small liver malignancies. One of the largest series revealed that there is only a 1.8% early recurrence rate within 15 months in primary and metastatic liver tumors. Further, RFA for small HCC < 3 cm in size induced a near-complete necrosis rate of 90% at 6 months *(Table V)*; however, only about 67% of patients remained tumor-free during a 12- to 23-month follow-up [81, 82]. Results for metastatic liver tumors are slightly less promising with a 52% to 67% complete ablation rate at 1 year and survival rates of 96%, 64% and 40% at 1, 3, and 5 years, respectively [81, 83].

Electromagnetic waves from a needle electrode inserted at laparoscopy, laparotomy or percutaneously into the tumor are used for **microwave thermal ablation**. Response rates for patients with HCC were reported between 60% to 100% dependent on tumor size. Tumors 3 cm in diameter or smaller responded in more than 70% of cases compared with 53% in bigger tumors. Further, well, moderately and poorly differentiated HCCs responded in 85%, 25% and 0% of lesions. One and 2 year survival rates of 83% and 69% can be achieved [72].

Table V. 5-year survival after radiofrequency ablation for HCC in series since 1990

Author	Reference	Year	No. of patients	Patient survival (%)			Tumor
				1 year	3 years	5 years	
Rossi et al.	[95]	1996	39	94	68	40	HCC*[1]
Buscarini et al.	[96]	2001	88	89	62	33	HCC

* Tumor size was ≤ 3.5 cm. [1] HCC : hepatocellular carcinoma.

Low-power laser energy can be applied percutaneously with thin fiber-optic fibers. After single sessions of **laser-induced interstitial thermotherapy** (LITT), HCC nodules ranging from 10 to 66 mm in size underwent total necrosis in 82% of cirrhotic patients [72]. LITT performed under MRI guidance results in precise and reproducible areas of induced necrosis with a local control rate of up to 94% in various liver tumors, and with an improved survival rate. Thus, thermal ablation contributes to a remarkable local tumor control rate and improves survival [72, 74, 81, 84].

Gene therapy

To date about 10 clinical trials with a small number of patients have been performed for treatment of HCC in the USA, Egypt, UK and Spain with tumor-suppressor gene transfer, immunogenic therapy, suicide gene therapy and transfer of oncolytic viruses. Some of these patients treated for HCC have shown a tumor response with reduction of tumor volume and decrease of the AFP levels; however, data on clinical outcome of these patients are not available yet [85]. For metastatic tumors to the liver, few phase I and II trials have been conducted. Since both number of patients and results of treatment are limited, at present, the use of gene therapy is likely to be adjuvant therapy in combination with others [86].

Radiation

Most recently stereotactic single dose irradiation has been evaluated in a phase II study as a new approach for therapy of non-resectable liver metastases. In this prospective single center study metastases derived from colorectal carcinomas, breast cancer, sarcomas, bronchial cancer, pancreatic carcinomas and others in 47%, 26%, 9%, 6%, 5% and 7% of lesions, respectively. There were no major side effects and actuarial local tumor control was 82% after 1.5 year. Further, in patients without extrahepatic tumor manifestation survival was significantly higher compared with patients treated with a palliative intention (87% vs 24% after 1.5 year; $p < 0.001$) [87]. Gores et al. used a neoadjuvant protocol with external beam irradiation plus bolus 5-FU therapy followed by brachytherapy and protracted venous infusion of 5-FU for CCC before transplantation. With a mean follow-up of 41 months, in only about 8% of cases tumor recurrence occurred [1].

References

1. Kadry Z, Malekkiani N, Clavien PA. Treatment of primary and secondary liver malignancy. *Swiss Med Wkly* 2001; 131: 338-45.
2. Buell JF, Koffron A, Yoshida A, Hanway M, Lo A, Layman R, Cronin DC, Posner MC, Millis JM. Is any method of vascular control superior in hepatic resection of metastatic cancers? *Arch Surg* 2001; 136: 569-75.
3. Matsumata T, Ikeda Y, Hayashi H, Kamakura T, Taketomi A, Sugimachi K. The association between transfusion and cancer-free survival after curative resection for hepatocellular carcinoma. *Cancer* 1993; 72: 1866-71.
4. Redaelli CA, Dufour JF, Wagner M, Schilling M, Hüsler J, Krähenbühl L, Büchler MW, Reichen J. Preoperative galactose elimination capacity predicts complications and survival after hepatic resection. *Ann Surg* 2002; 235: 77-85.
5. Redaelli CA, Wagner M, Krähenbühl L, Gloor B, Schilling MK, Dufour JF, Büchler. Liver surgery in the era of tissue-preserving resections: early and late outcome in patients with primary and secondary hepatic tumors. *World J Surg* 2002; 26: 1126-32.
6. Savage PA, Malt AR. Survival after hepatic resection for malignant tumours. *Br J Surg* 1992; 79: 1095-101.
7. Jaeck D, Bachellier PGM, Boudjema K, Vaillant JC, Balladur P, Nordlinger B. Long-term survival following resection of colorectal hepatic metastases. *Br J Surg* 1997; 84: 977-80.
8. Lehnert T, Otto G, Herfarth C. Therapeutic modalities and prognostic factors in primary and secondary liver tumors. *World J Surg* 1995; 19: 252-63.
9. Doci R, Gennari L, Bignami P, Montalto F, Morabito A, Bozzetti F, Bonalumi MG. Morbidity and mortality after hepatic resection of metastases from colorectal cancer. *Br J Surg* 1995; 82: 377-81.
10. Hollbrook RF, Koo K, Ryan JA. Resection of malignant primary tumors. *Am J Surg* 1996; 171: 453-5.
11. Zibari GB, Rich A, Zizzi HC, *et al*. Surgical and nonsurgical management of primary and metastatic liver tumors. *Am Surg* 1998; 64: 211-20.
12. Nagorney DM, Van der Heerden JA, Ilstrup DM, Adson MA. Primary hepatic malignancy: surgical management and determinants of survival. *Surgery* 1989; 106: 740-9.
13. Kanematsu T, Furui J, Yanaga K, Okudaira S, Shimada M, Shirabe K. A 16-year experience in performing hepatic resection in 303 patients with hepatocellular carcinoma: 1995-2000. *Surgery* 2002; 131: 153-8.
14. The terminology committee of the IHPBA. The Brisbane 2000 terminology of hepatic anatomy and resections. *HPB* 2000; 2: 333-9.
15. Liu CL, Fan ST, Lo CM, Tung-Ping Poon R, Wong J. Anterior approach for major hepatic resection for large hepatocellular carcinoma. *Ann Surg* 2000; 232: 25-9.
16. Yamamoto J, Kosuge T, Shimada K, Yamasaki S. Anterior approach for isolated resection of the caudate lobe of the liver. *World J Surg* 1999; 23: 97-102.
17. Weitz J, Koch M, Kienle P, Schrodel A, Herfarth C. Detection of hematogenic tumor cell dissemination in patients undergoing resection of liver metastases of colorectal cancer. *Ann Surg* 2000; 232: 66-71.
18. Lai ECS, Fan ST, Lo CM, Chu KM, Liu CL. Anterior approach for difficult major right hepatectomy. *World J Surg* 1996; 20: 314-8.
19. Gerhards MF, van Gulik TM, de Wit LT, Obertop H, Gouma DJ. Evaluation of morbidity and mortality after resection for hilar cholangiocarcinoma – a single center experience. *Surgery* 2000; 127: 395-400.
20. Kosuge T, Yamamoto J, Shimada K, Yamasaki S, Makuuchi M. Improved surgical results for hilar cholangiocarcinoma with procedures including major hepatic resection. *Ann Surg* 1999; 230: 663-5.
21. Neuhaus P, Jonas S, Bechstein WO, Lohmann R, *et al*. Extended resections for hilar cholangiocarcinoma. *Ann Surg* 1999; 230: 808-12.

22. Todoroki T, Kawamoto T, Koike N, Takahashi H, *et al.* Radical resection of hilar bile duct carcinoma and predictors of survival. *Br J Surg* 2000; 87: 306-9.
23. Nagino M, Kamiya J, Uesaka K, Sano T, Yamamoto H, Hayakawa N, Kanai M, Nimura Y. Complications of hepatectomy for hilar cholangiocarcinoma. *World J Surg* 2001; 25: 1277-83.
24. Alessiani M, Tzakis A, Todo S, Demetris AJ. Assessment of five-year experience with abdominal cluster transplantation. *J Am Coll Surg* 1995; 180: 1.
25. Neuhaus SJ, Texler M, Hewett PJ, Watson D. Port-site metastases following laparoscopic surgery. *Br J Surg* 1998; 85: 735-41.
26. Poulin EC, Mamazza J, Schlachta CM, Gregoire R, Roy N. Laparoscopic resection does not adversely affect survival curves in patients undergoing surgery for colorectal adenocarcinoma. *Ann Surg* 1995; 229: 487-92.
27. Cherqui D, Husson E, Hammond R, Malassagne B, Stéphan F, Bensaid S, Rotman N, Fagniez PL. Laparoscopic liver resections: a feasibility study in 30 patients. *Ann Surg* 2000; 232: 753-62.
28. Watanabe Y, Sato M, Ueda S, *et al.* Laparoscopic hepatic resection: a new safe procedure by abdominal wall lifting method. *Hepatogastroenterol* 1997; 44: 143-7.
29. Moskop RJ, Lubarsky DA. Carbon dioxide embolism during laparoscopic cholecystectomy. *South Med J* 1994; 84: 414-5.
30. Schlitt HJ, Oldhafer KJ, Bornscheuer A, Pichlmayr R. *In situ*, *ante situm*, and *ex situ* surgical approaches for otherwise irresectable hepatic tumors. *Acta Chir Austriaca* 1998; 30: 215-8.
31. Oldhafer KJ, Lang H, Schlitt HJ, Hauss J, *et al.* Long-term experience after *ex situ* liver surgery. *Surgery* 2000; 127: 520-6.
32. Raab R, Schlitt HJ, Oldhafer KJ, Bornscheuer A, *et al.* Ex vivo resection techniques in tissue-preserving surgery for liver malignancies. *Langenbecks Arch Chir* 2000; 385: 179-84.
33. Yamanaka N, Takata T, Yamanaka J, Jasui C, Ando T, Maeda S, Okamoto E. Evolution of and obstacles in surgical treatment for hepatocellular carcinoma over the last 25 years: differences over four treatment eras. *J Gastroenterol* 1990; 35: 613-21.
34. Nagasue N, Yamanoi A, et-Assal ON, Ohmori H, Tachibana M, Kimoto T, Kohno H. Major compared with limited hepatic resection for hepatocellular carcinoma without underlying cirrhosis: a retrospective analysis. *Eur J Surg* 1999; 165: 638-46.
35. Takenaka K, Yamamoto K, Takatomi A, Itasaka H, Adachi E, Shirabe K, Nishizaki T, Yanaga K, Sugimachi K. A comparison of the surgical results in patients with hepatitis B *versus* hepatitis C-related hepatocellular carcinoma. *Hepatology* 1995; 22: 20-4.
36. Lai EC, Fan ST, Lo CM, Chu KM, Liu CL, Wong J. Hepatic resection for hepatocellular carcinoma. An audit of 343 patients. *Ann Surg* 1995; 221: 291-8.
37. Hanazaki K, Kajikawa S, Shimozawa N, Mihara M, Shimada K, Hiraguri M, Koike N, Adachi W, Amano J. Survival and recurrence after hepatic resection of 386 consecutive patients with hepatocellular carcinoma. *J Am Coll Surg* 2000; 191: 381-8.
38. Lillemoe KD, Cameron JLCJL. Surgery for hilar cholangiocarcinoma: the Johns Hopkins approach. *J Hepatobiliary Pancreat Surg* 2000; 7: 115-21.
39. Lee S, Lee YJ, Park KM, Hwang S, Min PC. One hundred and eleven liver resections for hilar bile duct cancer. *J Hepatobiliary Pancreat Surg* 2000; 7: 135-41.
40. Scheele J, Stangl R, Altendorf-Hofmann A, Gall FP. Indicators of prognosis after hepatic resection for colorectal secondaries. *Surgery* 1991; 110: 13-29.
41. Rosen CB, Nagorney DM, Taswell HF, Helgeson SL, Iistrup DM, van Heerden JA, Adson MA. Perioperative blood transfusion and determinants of survival after liver resection for metastatic colorectal carcinoma. *Ann Surg* 1992; 216: 493-505.
42. Gayowski T, Iwatsuki S, Madariaga JR, Selby R, Todo S, Irish W, Starzl TE, Hafner GH. Experience in hepatic resection for metastatic colorectal cancer: analysis of clinical and pathological risk factors. *Surgery* 1994; 116: 703-10.

43. Scheele J, Stangl R, Altendorf-Hofmann A, *et al.* Resection of colorectal liver metastases. *World J Surg* 1995; 19: 59-71.
44. Nordlinger B, Guiguet M, Vaillant JC, *et al.* Surgical resection of colorectal carcinoma metastases to the liver. A prognostic scoring system to improve case selection, based on 1,568 patients. *Cancer* 1996; 77: 1254-62.
45. Jamison RL, Donohue JH, Nagorney DM, *et al.* Hepatic resection for colorectal cancer results in cure for some patients. *Arch Surg* 1997; 132: 505-10.
46. Bakalakos EA, Kim JA, Young DC, Martin EW. Determinants of survival following hepatic resection for metastatic colorectal cancer. *World J Surg* 1998; 22: 399-404.
47. Fong Y, Fortner J, Sun RL, Brennan MF, Blumgart LH. Clinical score for predicting recurrence after hepatic resection for metastatic colorectal cancer: analysis of 1,001 consecutive cases. *Ann Surg* 1999; 230: 309-18.
48. Iwatsuki S, Dvorchik I, Madariaga JR, *et al.* Hepatic resection for metastatic colorectal adenocarcinoma: a proposal of a prognostic scoring system. *J Am Coll Surg* 1999; 189: 291-9.
49. Pichlmayr R, Weimann A, Ringe B. Indications for liver transplantation in hepatobiliary malignancy. *Hepatology* 1994; 20: 33-40.
50. Penn I. Hepatic transplantation for primary and metastatic cancer of the liver. *Surgery* 1991; 110: 726-34.
51. Iwatsuki S, Dvorchik I, Marsh JW, Madariaga JR, Carr B, Fung JJ. Liver transplantation for hepatocellular carcinoma: a proposal of a prognostic scoring system. *J Am Coll Surg* 2000; 191: 389-94.
52. Colella G, De Cartis L, Rondinara GF, Sansalone CV, Belli LS, Aseni A, *et al.* Is hepatocellular carcinoma in cirrhosis an actual indication for liver transplantation. *Transplant Proc* 1997; 29: 492-4.
53. Figueras J, Jaurrieta E, Valls C, Ramos E, Sorrano T, Rafecas A, *et al.* Resection or transplantation for hepatocellular carcinoma in cirrhotic patients: outcomes based on indicated treatment strategy. *J Am Coll Surg* 2000; 190: 580-7.
54. Tamura S, Kato T, Berho M, Misiakos EP, O'Brian CA, Reddy KR, *et al.* Impact of histological grade of hepatocellular carcinoma on the outcome of liver transplantation. *Arch Surg* 2001; 136: 25-30.
55. Jones S, Bechstein WO, Steinmüller T, Herrmann M, Radke C, Berg T, *et al.* Vascular invasion and histopathologic grading determine outcome after liver transplantation. *Hepatology* 2001; 33: 25-30.
56. O'Grady J, Polson RJ, Rolles K, Calne RY, Williams R. Liver transplantation for malignant disease. *Ann Surg* 1988; 207: 373-9.
57. Pichlmayr R, Weimann A, Klempnauer J, Oldhafer KJ, Maschek H, Tusch G, Ringe B. Surgical treatment in proximal bile duct cancer: a single center experience. *Ann Surg* 1996; 224: 628-38.
58. Casavilla A, Marsh JW, Iwatsuki S, Todo S, Lee RG, Madariaga JR, *et al.* Hepatic resection and transplantation for peripheral cholangiocarcinoma. *J Am Coll Surg* 1997; 185: 429-36.
59. Iwatsuki S, Todo S, Marsh JW, Madariaga JR, Lee RG, Dvorchik I, *et al.* Treatment of hilar cholangiocarcinoma (Klatskin tumors) with hepatic resection or transplantation. *J Am Coll Surg* 1998; 187: 358-64.
60. Devlin J, O'Grady J. Indications for referral and assessment in adult liver transplantation: a clinical guideline. *Gut* 1999; 45 (Suppl. 6): 1-22.
61. Wall WJ, Marotta PJ. Surgery and transplantation for hepatocellular cancer. *Liver Transpl* 2000; 6: S16-S22.
62. Klintmalm GB. Liver transplantation for hepatocellular carcinoma. A registry report of the impact of tumor characteristics on outcome. *Ann Surg* 1998; 228: 479-90.
63. Wakabayashi H, Ishimura K, Okano K, Izuishi K, Karasawa Y, Goda F, Maeba T, Maeta H. Is preoperative portal vein embolization effective in improving prognosis after major hepatic resection in patients with advanced-stage hepatocellular carcinoma? *Cancer* 2001; 92: 2384-90.

64. Tanaka H, Hirohashi K, Kubo S, Higashi I, Kinoshita H. Preoperative portal vein embolization improves prognosis after right hepatectomy for hepatocellular carcinoma in patients with impaired hepatic function. *Br J Surg* 2000; 87: 879-82.
65. Abdalla EK, Hicks M, Vauthery JN. Portal vein embolization: rationale, technique and future prospects. *Br J Surg* 2001; 88: 165-9.
66. Azoulay D, Castaing D, Smail A, Adam R. Resection of nonresectable liver metastases from colorectal cancer after percutaneous portal vein embolization. *Ann Surg* 2000; 231: 480-6.
67. de Baere T, Roche A, Elias D, Lasser P, *et al*. Preoperative portal vein embolization for extension of hepatectomy indications. *Hepatology* 1996; 24: 1386-91.
68. Lorenz M, Schramm H, Gassel HJ, *et al*. Randomized trial of surgery *versus* surgery followed by adjuvant hepatic arterial infusion with 5-fluorouracil and folinic acid for liver metastases of colorectal cancer. *Ann Surg* 1998; 228: 756-9.
69. Kemeny N, Huang Y, Cohen AM, Shi W, *et al*. Hepatic arterial infusion of chemotherapy after resection of hepatic metastases from colorectal cancer. *N Engl J Med* 1999; 341: 2039-43.
70. Bismuth H, Adam R, Levi F, Farabos C, *et al*. Resection of nonresectable liver metastases from colorectal cancer after neoadjuvant chemotherapy. *Ann Surg* 1996; 224: 509-12.
71. Giacchetti S, Itzhaki M, Gruia G, Adam R, *et al*. Long-term survival of patients with unresectable colorectal cancer liver metastases following infusional chemotherapy with 5-fluorouracil, leucovorin, oxaliplatin and surgery. *Ann Oncol* 1999; 10: 663-6.
72. Alsowmely AM, Hodgson HJF. Review article: non-surgical treatment of hepatocellular carcinoma. *Aliment Pharmacol Ther* 2002; 16: 1-15.
73. Sotsky TK, Ravikumar TS. Cryotherapy in the treatment of liver metastases from colorectal cancer. *Semin Oncol* 2002; 29: 183-91.
74. Pimrose JN. Treatment of colorectal metastases: surgery, cryotherapy, or radiofrequency ablation. *Gut* 2002; 50: 1-5.
75. Befeler AS, Di Bisceglie AM. Hepatocellular carcinoma: diagnosis and treatment. *Gastroenterology* 2002; 122: 1609-19.
76. Giovannini M. Percutaneous alcohol ablation for liver metastasis. *Semin Oncol* 2002; 29: 192-5.
77. Dick EA, Taylor-Robinson SD, Thomas HC, Gedroyc WMW. Ablative therapy for liver tumours. *Gut* 2001; 50: 733-9.
78. Weinreich DM, Alexander HR. Transarterial perfusion of liver metastases. *Semin Oncol* 2002; 29: 136-44.
79. Dizon DS, Kemeny N. Intrahepatic arterial infusion of chemotherapy: clinical results. *Semin Oncol* 2002; 29: 126-35.
80. Sullivan KL. Hepatic artery chemoembolization. *Semin Oncol* 2002; 29: 145-51.
81. Wood BJ, Ramkaransingh JR, Fojo T, Walther MM, Libutti SK. Percutaneous tumor ablation with radiofrequency. *Cancer* 2002; 94: 443-51.
82. Allgaier HP, Galandi D, Zuber I, Blum HE. Radiofrequency thermal ablation of hepatocellular carcinoma. *Dig Dis* 2002; 19: 301-10.
83. Parikh AA, Curley SA, Fornage BD, Ellis LM. Radiofrequency ablation of hepatic metastases. *Semin Oncol* 2002; 29: 168-82.
84. Kuyvenhoven JP, Lamers CBHW, van Hoek B. Practical management of hepatocellular carcinoma. *Scand J Gastroenterol* 2001; 36: 82-7.
85. Ruiz J, Mazzolini G, Sangro B, Qian C, Prieto J. Gene therapy of hepatocellular carcinoma. *Dig Dis* 2001; 19: 324-32.
86. Havlik R, Jiao LR, Nicholls J, Jensen SL, Habib NA. Gene therapy for liver metastases. *Semin Oncol* 2002; 29: 202-8.
87. Herfarth KK, Debus J, Lohr F, Bahner ML, Wannenmacher M. Stereotaktische Bestrahlung von Lebermetastasen. *Der Radiologe* 2001; 41: 64-8.

88. Bronowicki JP, Vetter D, Dumas D, *et al.* Transcatheter oily chemoembolization for hepatocellular carcinoma. A 4-year study of 127 French patients. *Cancer* 1994; 47: 16-24.
89. Stefanini GF, Amorati P, Biselli M, *et al.* Efficacy of transarterial targeted treatments on survival of patients with hepatocellular carcinoma: an Italian experience. *Cancer* 1995; 75: 2427-34.
90. Groupe d'Étude et de Traitement du Carcinome Hepatocellulaire. A comparison of lipiodol chemoembolization and conservative treatment for unresectable hepatocellular carcinoma. *N Engl J Med* 1995; 332: 1256-61.
91. Pelletier G, Ducreux M, Gay F, *et al.* Treatment of unresectable hepatocellular carcinoma with lipiodol chemoembolization: multicenter randomized trial. *J Hepatol* 1998; 29: 129-34.
92. Shiina S, Tagawa K, Niwa Y, *et al.* Percutaneous ethanol injection therapy for hepatocellular carcinoma: results in 146 patients. *Am J Roentgenol* 1993; 160: 1023-8.
93. Lencioni R, Bartolozzi C, Caramella D, *et al.* Treatment for small hepatocellular carcinoma with percutaneous ethanol injection. Analysis of prognostic factors in 105 western patients. *Cancer* 1995; 76: 1737-46.
94. Livraghi T, Giorgio A, Marin G, *et al.* Hepatocellular carcinoma and cirrhosis in 746 patients: long-term results of percutaneous ethanol injection. *Radiology* 1995; 197: 101-8.
95. Rossi S, Di Stasi M, Buscardini E, *et al.* Percutaneous RF interstitial thermal ablation in the treatment of hepatic cancer. *Am J Roentgenol* 1996; 167: 759-68.
96. Buscarini L, Buscarini E, Di Stasi M, *et al.* Percutaneous radiofrequency ablation of small hepatocellular carcinoma: long-term results. *Eur Radiol* 2001; 11: 914-21.

Prevention of hepatocellular carcinoma

Thierry Poynard, Vlad Ratziu

Service d'Hépato-Gastroentérologie, Groupe Hospitalier Pitié-Salpêtrière, Paris, France

Hepatocellular carcinoma (HCC), the most frequent cause of primary liver cancer, occurs almost exclusively in patients with chronic liver disease, extensive fibrosis or cirrhosis [1-9]. There is no very effective treatment of hepatocellular carcinoma but there are several very effective treatments of chronic liver diseases. More advances have been made in the prevention of cirrhosis than in the prevention of hepatocellular carcinoma in patients with cirrhosis [5].

Therefore the present best strategy to prevent hepatocellular carcinoma is the prevention of chronic liver disease or the decrease of fibrosis progression. The aim of this text is to review the treatments effective in reducing fibrosis progression or hepatocellular carcinoma occurrence. The knowledge of factors associated with fibrosis progression and hepatocellular carcinoma occurrence could permit to optimise screening and treatment strategies [10, 11].

Target of prevention: chronic liver diseases

The largest populations at risk of HCC are patients infected by hepatitis B virus, hepatitis C virus, patients with high alcohol consumption, patients with insulin-resistance (overweight, diabetes, dyslipidemia), and genetic hemochromatosis *(Table I)*.

The worldwide prevalence of patients at risk of liver fibrosis and cirrhosis is therefore huge, around 1 billion people. The estimated mortality due to cirrhosis is 779,000 and to hepatocellular carcinoma 501,000; with 1,280,000 annual deaths, fibrotic liver is the eighth cause of mortality in the world [7]. The incidence of hepatocellular carcinoma is rising globally, due largely to the epidemic spread of HCV infection. Several factors are associated with fibrosis progression that varies between chronic liver diseases. For example,

Table I. Population at risk of liver fibrosis, cirrhosis and hepatocellular carcinoma

Liver fibrosis risk factor	Worldwide prevalence (n)	Age of cirrhosis 50th percentile (years)	
		Male	Female
Insulin-resistance: diabetes, overweight, dyslipidemia	10% (600,000,000)	Unknown	Unknown
High alcohol consumption	10% (600,000,000)	61	61
Hepatitis B virus chronic infection	5% (300,000,000)	65	67
Hepatitis C virus chronic infection	3% (180,000,000)	69	74
Genetic hemochromatosis	0.5% (30,000,000)	66	78

the highest fibrosis progression rate is observed in patients coinfected with HIV and HCV with occurrence of cirrhosis and hepatocellular carcinoma 15 to 20 years before patients infected by HCV alone [10].

Treatments effective in reducing liver fibrosis progression and cirrhosis occurrence

Hepatitis C

Factors associated with fibrosis progression

Factors associated and not associated with fibrosis are summarised in *Table II*. Several factors have been clearly shown to be associated with fibrosis progression rate [10, 12-17]: duration of infection, age, male gender, alcohol consumption, HIV coinfection and low CD4 count. The progression from infection to cirrhosis depends strongly on sex and age. Age and duration of infection were found to be significant independent cofactors of progression. The female gender is associated to less rapid progression to cirrhosis than male whatever the age. Metabolic factors (diabetes, insulin-resistance, overweight) seem also to be associated with more rapid fibrosis progression.

Table II. Factors associated or not with fibrosis progression in chronic hepatitis C

Associated in uni and multivariate analysis	Not sure	Not associated
Age at infection	Necrosis	Last serum viral load
Duration of infection	Inflammation	Genotype
Age at biopsy	Hemochromatosis heterozygote	Mode of infection
Consumption of alcohol > 50g per day	Cigarette consumption	DR antigens
HIV coinfection	Steatosis	Liver viral load
CD4 count < 200/ml	Body Mass Index	HCV-HVR1 complexity
Male gender	Moderate alcohol consumption	
Fibrosis stage	Glucose intolerance	

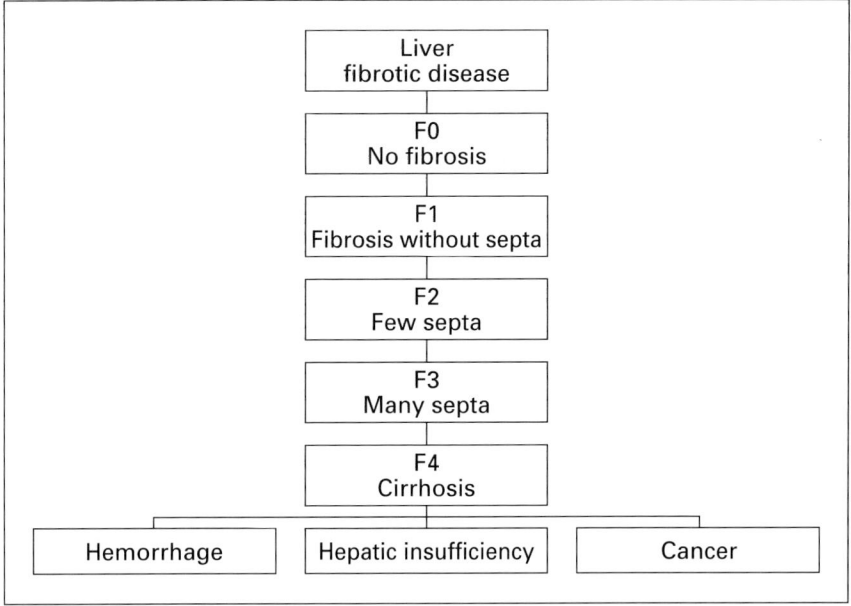

Figure 1. The model of fibrosis progression in chronic liver disease. Estimated key numbers of fibrosis natural history from literature and our database: the median time from infection (F0) to cirrhosis (F4) is 30 years. The mortality at 10 years for cirrhosis is 50%. The transition probability per year from non-complicated cirrhosis to each of the complications is around 3%. Main factors associated with fibrosis progression are age and gender, whatever the cause of liver fibrosis.

Impact of treatment on fibrosis progression

Several studies have demonstrated the impact on fibrosis progression of different regimens in patients with chronic hepatitis C [17-20].

According to a Markov age-dependent modelling, a ten-year increment in duration of infection increased the risk of progression by 32% for IFN-treated patients and by 51% for untreated patients. The course of a series of 1,000 IFN-treated and 1,000 untreated patients was simulated over 5 years according to the initial stage of fibrosis and age and duration of infection at diagnosis. IFN treatment decreased the risk of progression to F3+F4 by a factor of 4.8, for subjects aged 40 years, infected for 10 years, and in F0+F1 at diagnosis. As age and duration of infection increased, the risk of fibrosis increased and the impact of IFN treatment decreased.

We pooled individual data from 3,010 naïve patients with pre-treatment and post-treatment biopsies from 4 randomised trials [20]. Ten different regimens combining standard interferon, PEG interferon, and ribavirin were compared. The impact of each regimen was estimated by the percentage of patients with at least 1 grade improvement in the necrosis and inflammation (METAVIR score), the percentage of patients with at least 1 stage worsening in fibrosis METAVIR score, and by the fibrosis progression rate per year. Necrosis and inflammation improvement ranged from 39% (interferon 24 weeks) to 73% (PEG 1.5 (g/kg + ribavirin >10.6mg/kg/day; $p < 0.001$). Fibrosis worsening ranges from

23% (interferon 24 weeks) to 8% (PEG 1.5 (g/kg + ribavirin >10.6mg/kg/day; $p < 0.001$). All regimens significantly reduced the fibrosis progression rates in comparison to rates before treatment. The reversal of cirrhosis was observed in 75 patients (49%) of 153 patients with baseline cirrhosis.

Six factors were independently associated with the absence of significant fibrosis after treatment: baseline fibrosis stage (odds ration [OR] = 0.12; $p < 0.0001$), sustained viral response (OR = 0.36; $p < 0.0001$), age < 40 years (OR = 0.51; $p < 0.001$), body mass index < 27 kg/m2 (OR = 0.65; $p < 0.001$), no or minimal baseline activity (OR = 0.70; $p = 0.02$), and viral load < 3.5 millions copies per millilitre (OR = 0.79; $p = 0.03$).

Impact of treatment on hepatocellular carcinoma occurrence and mortality

There is an obvious ethical problem in conducting large randomised trials comparing treatment of chronic hepatitis C (very effective on virological and histological endpoints) with placebo in order to prove the reduction of mortality [21]. Retrospective studies controlled or not have shown a decrease in morbidity and mortality in patients treated with interferon [21-29]. The reduction in mortality is significant in patients without sustained virologic response (OR=0.47; p=0.002) but is higher in patients with a sustained virologic response (OR=0.15; p=0.0001) and in non-cirrhotic patients (OR=0.36; p=0.02) [23].

Hepatitis B

Factors associated with fibrosis progression

There is little information concerning the annual rate of development of cirrhosis in chronic HBV carriers as well as risk factors associated with the fibrosis progression rate [28-32]. However several similar factors have been identified: age, coinfection with HIV, and alcohol consumption [11]. Factors associated and not associated with cirrhosis or hepatocellular carcinoma are summarised in *Table III*.

Impact of treatment on fibrosis progression

As in hepatitis C many progresses have been made in the management of patients with hepatitis B.

There are two approved regimens, interferon and lamivudine with two products close to approval, adefovir and Pegylated interferons [28-42]. Interferon, lamivudine and adefovir have demonstrated their efficacy in reducing necrosis and fibrosis [34-36]. However, there are far less trials than in hepatitis C studies with fewer evaluations of treatment impact on fibrosis progression rate and of associated factors.

Interferon alpha achieves a short-term outcome of around 20-30% loss of HBeAg *versus* 5% to 10% without treatment. The efficacy is lower in Chinese patients, who are immunotolerant to HBV because of acquisition of the disease during early childhood, than in white patients. This difference is further confirmed on long-term follow-up. Interferon alpha probably does not affect the development of cirrhosis-related complications in

Table III. Factors associated with progression to cirrhosis or to cancer in HBV carriers

Factors	Cirrhosis	Hepatocellular carcinoma
Age at infection	Yes	Yes
Duration of infection	yes	Yes
Male gender	Yes	Yes
Age at biopsy	Yes	Yes
Consumption of alcohol > 50g per day	Yes	Yes
HCV coinfection	Yes	Not sure
Delta coinfection	Yes	Not sure
CD4 count < 200/ml	Yes	Not sure
Fibrosis stage	Yes	Yes
Necrosis	Not sure	Not sure
Inflammation	Not sure	Not sure
Genotype	Not sure	Not sure
Pre-core mutant	Not sure	Not sure
Core-promoter mutant	Not sure	Not sure
Sero conversion anti-HBe	Not sure	Not sure
HBV-DNA level	Not sure	Not sure
Aflatoxin	Not sure	Yes

Table IV. Treatments associated with decrease of liver fibrosis progression or decrease of hepatocellular carcinoma incidence

Factors	Liver fibrosis progression	Hepatocellular carcinoma
HBV infection		
HBV vaccination	Yes	Yes
Interferon	Yes	Yes
Lamivudine	Yes	Unknown
Adefovir	Yes	Unknown
HCV infection		
Interferon	Yes	Yes
Interferon-ribavirin	Yes	Unknown
PEG interferon	Yes	Unknown
PEG-interferon-ribavirin	Yes	Unknown
Alcoholic liver disease		
Alcohol consumption reduction	Yes	Yes
Colchicine	No	No
Silymarin	No	No
Hemochromatosis		
Phlebotomy	Yes	Yes
Metabolic disease		
Diabetes-insulin resistance treatment	Unknown	Unknown
Weight reduction	Unknown	Unknown

Chinese patients, whereas in white patients, the frequency of long-term complications is reduced if interferon alpha is successful in inducing loss of HBeAg.

Lamivudine profoundly suppresses viral replication and achieves an HBeAg seroconversion rate similar to that of interferon alpha. It is equally effective in Chinese and white patients because the main antiviral mechanism is through inhibition of reverse transcription of HBV during viral replication. However, long-term lamivudine therapy is associated with emergence of HBV variants, YMDD variants.

There are few comparisons between lamivudine, interferon or lamivudine interferon combination [37, 38]. Trials of combinations of PEG interferon and lamivudine, adefovir or other nucleosides are needed.

Adefovir at the dose of 10 mg is effective and safe and is not associated with emergence of HBV variants, at least at two years follow-up [39-41].

Vaccination and prevention of hepatocellular carcinoma

Universal vaccination program is the best-proved preventive treatment of hepatitis B complications, including cancer, recommended by WHO since 1991 [43-48]. The cost benefit is higher in areas of low, intermediate and high endemicity. In countries of very low endemicity, economic evaluations have yielded contradictory results, depending on the type of epidemiological model they used. The cost-effectiveness of adding universal to selective vaccination strategies in these countries depends on the selective strategies' ability to sufficiently identify, reach and fully vaccinate persons in various risk groups.

In Western countries as in France, a controversy exists about the risk of demyelinating diseases after hepatitis B vaccination [49]. The results of several controlled studies indicate no significant association between hepatitis B vaccination and the development of demyelinating diseases including multiple sclerosis [49-53]. Despite the absence of significant proofs, the prevalence of vaccination has decreased from 90% to 30% in French infants in the last 5 years. Even a worst scenario against vaccination demonstrates the benefit of vaccination. If the risk of 0.24 demyelinating diseases per 100,000 hepatitis B vaccinations was true (highest prediction), a total of 1.9 case will appear out of 800,000 children *versus* (lowest predictions) 3 fulminant hepatitis B, 60 chronic hepatitis B and 12 hepatocellular carcinomas.

Other chronic liver disease

Very few studies have been made in other chronic liver diseases.

In alcoholic liver disease, the only effective treatment is alcohol abstinence [54-58]. No treatment has clearly proven a decrease in fibrosis progression or in hepatocellular carcinoma incidence. In non-alcoholic steato-hepatitis and fibrosis associated with metabolic diseases (insulin resistance, diabetes, overweight), there is so far no effective treatment [59].

In hemochromatosis despite the absence of randomized trials several studies have demonstrated that early diagnosis and phlebotomy therapy largely prevent the adverse consequences of iron overload [60, 61]. The prognosis of hemochromatosis and most of its complications, including liver cancer, depends on the amount and duration of iron excess. Patients adequately treated with phlebotomy had a higher survival than inadequately treated patients. Adequately treated patients with cirrhosis and/or diabetes had better survival than inadequately treated patients with similar organ damage. Adequate phlebotomy treatment is the major determinant of survival and markedly improved prognosis.

Conclusion

The most effective prevention of hepatocellular carcinoma is the prevention of liver fibrotic diseases. There are nowadays very effective treatments of frequent chronic liver diseases *(Table IV)*: vaccination, interferon, lamivudine and adefovir for hepatitis B; pegylated interferon and ribavirin for hepatitis C; phlebotomy for hemochromatosis. Diagnosis of extensive fibrosis before cirrhosis stage by non-invasive biochemical markers should improve screening strategies [62].

References

1. Montalto G, Cervello M, Giannitrapani L, Dantona F, Terranova A, Castagnetta LA. Epidemiology, risk factors, and natural history of hepatocellular carcinoma. *Ann N Y Acad Sci* 2002; 963: 13-20.
2. El-Serag HB, Mason A. Rising incidence of hepatocellular carcinoma in the United States. *N Engl J Med* 1999; 34: 745-50.
3. Chiaramonte M, Stroffolini T, Vian A, *et al.* Rate of incidence of hepatocellular carcinoma in patients with compensated viral cirrhosis. *Cancer* 1999; 85: 2132-7.
4. Takano S, Yokosuka O, Imazeki F, Tagawa M, Omata M. Incidence of hepatocellular carcinoma in chronic hepatitis B and C: a prospective study of 251 patients. *Hepatology* 1995; 21: 650-5.
5. Mast EE, Alter MJ, Margolis HS. Strategies to prevent and control hepatitis B and C virus infections: a global perspective. *Vaccine* 1999; 17: 1730-3.
6. W.H.O. Hepatitis C: global prevalence. *Wkly Epidemiol Rec* 1997; 72: 341-4.
7. Murray CJL, Lopez AD. Mortality by cause for eight regions of the world: Global Burden of Disease Study. *Lancet* 1997; 349: 1269-76.
8. Deuffic S, Buffat L, Poynard T, Valleron AJ. Modeling the hepatitis C virus epidemic in France. *Hepatology* 1999; 29: 1596-601.
9. Alter MJ, Kruszon-Moran D, Nainan OV, *et al.* The prevalence of hepatitis C virus infection in the United States, 1988 through 1994. *N Engl J Med* 1999; 341: 556-62.
10. Poynard T, Ratziu V, Charlotte F, Goodman Z, McHutchison J, Albrecht J. Rates and risk factors of liver fibrosis progression in patients with chronic hepatitis C. *J Hepatol* 2001; 34: 730-9.
11. Poynard T, Mathurin P, Lai CL, Guyader D, Poupon R, Tainturier MH, Myers RP, *et al.* A comparison of fibrosis progression in chronic liver diseases. *AASLD* 2001 (submitted).

12. Darby SC, Ewart DW, Giangrande PLF, *et al*. Mortality from liver cancer and liver disease in haemophilic men and boys given blood products contaminated with hepatitis C. *Lancet* 1997; 350: 1425-31.
13. Poynard T, Bedossa P, Opolon P, for the OBSVIRC, METAVIR, CLINIVIR and DOSVIRC groups. Natural history of liver fibrosis progression in patients with chronic hepatitis C. *Lancet* 1997; 349: 825-32.
14. Hourigan LF, MacDonald GA, Purdie D, Whitehall V, Shorthouse C, Clouston A, Powell EE. Fibrosis in chronic hepatitis C correlates significantly with body mass index and steatosis. *Hepatology* 1999; 29: 1215-9.
15. Hickman IJ, Clouston AD, Macdonald GA, Purdie DM, Prins JB, Ash S, Jonsson JR. Powell EE. Effect of weight reduction on liver histology and biochemistry in patients with chronic hepatitis C. *Gut* 2002; 51: 89-94.
16. Freeman AJ, Dore G, Law MG, Thorpe M, Overbeck JV, Lloyd AR, Marinos G, Kaldor JM. Estimating progression to cirrhosis in chronic hepatitis C virus infection. *Hepatology* 2001; 34: 809-16.
17. Deuffic-Burban S, Poynard T, Valleron AJ. Quantification of fibrosis progression in patients with chronic hepatitis C using a Markov model. *J Viral Hepat* 2002; 9: 114-22.
18. Sobesky R, Mathurin P, Charlotte F, *et al*. Modeling the impact of interferon alfa treatment on liver fibrosis progression in chronic hepatitis C: a dynamic view. *Gastroenterology* 1999; 116: 378-86.
19. Shiratori Y, Imazeki F, Moriyama M, *et al*. Histologic improvement of fibrosis in patients with hepatitis C who have sustained response to interferon therapy. *Ann Intern Med* 2000; 132: 517-24.
20. Poynard T, McHutchison J, Manns M, Trepo C, Lindsay K, Goodman Z, Ling MH, Albrecht J. Impact of pegylated interferon alfa-2b and ribavirin on liver fibrosis in patients with chronic hepatitis C. *Gastroenterology* 2002; 122: 1303-13.
21. Baffis V, Shrier I, Sherker AH, Szilagyi A. Use of interferon for prevention of hepatocellular carcinoma in cirrhotic patients with hepatitis B or hepatitis C virus infection. *Ann Intern Med* 1999; 131: 696-701.
22. Nishiguchi S, Kuroki T, Nakatani S, *et al*. Randomized trial of effects of Interferon alfa on incidence of hepatocellular carcinoma in chronic active hepatitis C with cirrhosis. *Lancet* 1995; 346: 1051-5.
23. Poynard T, Moussalli J, Ratziu V, *et al*. Is antiviral treatment (IFN alpha and/or ribavirin) justified in cirrhosis related to hepatitis C virus? Société Royale Belge de Gastro-entérologie. *Acta Gastroenterol Belg* 1998; 61: 431-7.
24. Yoshida H, Shiratori Y, Moriyama M, *et al*. Interferon therapy reduces the risk for hepatocellular carcinoma: national surveillance program of cirrhotic and non cirrhotic patients with chronic hepatitis C in Japan. *Ann Intern Med* 1999; 131: 174-81.
25. Yoshida H, Arakawa Y, Sata M, Nishiguchi S, Yano M, Fujiyama S, Yamada G, Yokosuka O, Shiratori Y, Omata M. Interferon therapy prolonged life expectancy among chronic hepatitis C patients. *Gastroenterology* 2002; 123: 483-91.
26. Dufour JF, DeLellis R, Kaplan MM. Regression of hepatic fibrosis in hepatitis C with long-term interferon treatment. *Dig Dis Sci* 1998; 43: 2573-6.
27. Bruno S, Battezzati PM, Bellati G, Manzin A, Maggioni M, Crosignani A, Borzio M, Solforosi L, Morabito A, Ideo G, Podda M. Long-term beneficial effects in sustained responders to interferon-alfa therapy for chronic hepatitis C. *J Hepatol* 2001; 34: 748-55.
28. Camma C, Giunta M, Andreone P, Craxi A. Interferon and prevention of hepatocellular carcinoma in viral cirrhosis: an evidence-based approach. *J Hepatol* 2001; 34: 593-602.
29. Maddrey WC. Hepatitis B: an important public health issue. *Clin Lab* 2001; 47: 51-5.
30. Sanchez-Tapias JM. Natural history of chronic hepatitis B. In: Buti M, Esteban R, Guardia J, eds. *Viral Hepatitis*. Barcelona: Accion Medica 2000: 21-31.
31. Lok ASF. Hepatitis B infection: pathogenesis and management. *J Hepatol* 2000; 32: 89-97.
32. Yuen MF, Lai CL. Treatment of chronic hepatitis B. *Lancet Infect Dis* 2001; 1: 232-41.

33. Yang HI, Lu SN, Liaw YF, You SL, Sun CA, Wang LY, Hsiao CK, Chen PJ, Chen DS, Chen CJ. Hepatitis B e antigen and the risk of hepatocellular carcinoma. *N Engl J Med* 2002 18; 347: 168-74.
34. Niederau C, Heintges T, Lange S, Goldmann G, Niederau CM, Mohr L, Haussinger D. Long-term follow-up of HBeAg-positive patients treated with interferon alfa for chronic hepatitis B. *N Engl J Med* 1996; 334: 1422-7.
35. Schiff ER, Heathcote J, Dienstag JL, *et al*. Improvements in liver histology and cirrhosis with extended lamivudine therapy. *Hepatology* 2000; 32: 296A.
36. Yao FY, Terrault NA, Freise C, Maslow L, Bass NM. Lamivudine treatment is beneficial in patients with severely decompensated cirrhosis and actively replicating hepatitis B infection awaiting liver transplantation: A comparative study using a matched, untreated cohort. *Hepatology* 2001; 34: 411-6.
37. Schalm SW, Heathcote J, Cianciara J, Farrell G, Sherman M, Willems B, *et al*. Lamivudine and alpha interferon combination treatment of patients with chronic hepatitis B infection: a randomised trial. *Gut* 2000; 46: 562-8.
38. Barbaro G, Zechini F, Pellicelli AM, Francavilla R, Scotto G, Bacca D, *et al*. Long-term efficacy of interferon alpha-2b and lamivudine in combination compared to lamivudine monotherapy in patients with chronic hepatitis B. An Italian multicenter, randomized trial. *J Hepatol* 2001; 35: 406-11.
39. Benhamou Y, Bochet M, Thibault V, Calvez V, Fievet MH, Vig P, Gibbs CS, Brosgart C, Fry J, Namini H, Katlama C, Poynard T. Safety and efficacy of adefovir dipivoxil in patients co-infected with HIV-1 and lamivudine-resistant hepatitis B virus: an open-label pilot study. *Lancet* 2001; 358: 718-23.
40. Marcellin P, Goodman Z, Chang TT, Lim SG, Tong M, Sievert W, Shiffman M, Jeffers L, Wulfsohn M, Fallis R, *et al*. Histological improvement in HBeAg positive chronic hepatitis B patients treated with adefovir dipivoxil. *J Hepatol* 2002; 36 (Suppl. 1): 8.
41. Hadziyannis S, Tassopolous N, Heathcote E, Chang TT, Kitis G, Rizzetto T, Marcellin P, Lim SG, Wulfsohn M, Wollman M, Fry J, Brosgart C. GS-98-438 a double blind, randomized, placebo-controlled study of adefovir dipivoxil (ADV) for presumed precore mutant chronic hepatitis B: 48 week results. *J Hepatol* 2002; 36 (Suppl. 1): 4.
42. Cooksley WGE, Piratvisuth T, Wang YJ, Mahachai V, Chao YC, Tanwandee T, Chutaputti A, Chang WY, Zahm FE, N. Pluck N. Evidence for the efficacy of peginterferon alfa-2a (40 KD) (PEGASYS) in the treatment of HBeAg-positive chronic hepatitis B (CHB) and impact of baseline factors. *J Hepatol* 2002; 36 (Suppl. 1): 8.
43. Prince AM. Perspectives on prophylactic and therapeutic immunization against hepatitis B and C viruses. *Transfus Clin Biol* 2001; 8: 467-70.
44. Chang MH, Shau WY, Chen CJ, Wu TC, Kong MS, Liang DC, Hsu HM, Chen HL, Hsu HY, Chen DS. Hepatitis B vaccination and hepatocellular carcinoma rates in boys and girls. *JAMA* 2000; 284: 3040-2.
45. Beutels P. Economic evaluations of hepatitis B immunization: a global review of recent studies (1994-2000). *Health Econ* 2001; 10: 751-74.
46. Stroffolini T, Mele A, Tosti ME, Gallo G, Balocchini E, Ragni P, *et al*. The impact of the hepatitis B mass immunisation campaign on the incidence and risk factors of acute hepatitis B in Italy. *J Hepatol* 2000; 33: 980-5.
47. Ni YH, Chang MH, Huang LM, Chen HL, Hsu HY, Chiu TY, *et al*. Hepatitis B virus infection in children and adolescents in a hyperendemic area: 15 years after mass hepatitis B vaccination. *Ann Intern Med* 2001; 135: 796-800.
48. Chang MH, Chen CJ, Lai MS, Hsu HM, Wu TC, Kong MS, *et al*. Universal hepatitis B vaccination in Taiwan and the incidence of hepatocellular carcinoma in children. Taiwan Childhood Hepatoma Study Group. *N Engl J Med* 1997; 336: 1855-9.
49. Cales P. Vaccination anti-hépatite B: modalités pratiques et histoire d'une polémique. *Hépato-Gastro* 2000; 7: 34-9.

50. Zipp F, Weil JG, Einhaupl KM. No increase in demyelinating diseases after hepatitis B vaccination. *Nat Med* 1999; 5: 964-5.
51. Sadovnick AD, Scheifele DW. School-based hepatitis B vaccination programme and adolescent multiple sclerosis. *Lancet* 2000; 355: 549-50.
52. Ascherio A, Zhang SM, Hernan MA, Olek MJ, Coplan PM, Brodovicz K, et al. Hepatitis B vaccination and the risk of multiple sclerosis. *N Engl J Med* 2001; 344: 327-32.
53. Confavreux C, Suissa S, Saddier P, Bourdes V, Vukusic S. Vaccinations and the risk of relapse in multiple sclerosis. Vaccines in Multiple Sclerosis Study Group. *N Engl J Med* 2001; 344: 319-26.
54. Diehl AM. Liver disease in alcohol abusers. Clinical perspective. *Alcohol* 2002; 27: 7-11.
55. Zureik M, Ducimetiere P. High alcohol-related premature mortality in France: concordant estimates from a prospective cohort study and national mortality statistics. *Alcohol Clin Exp Res* 1996; 20: 428-33.
56. Corrao G, Ferrari P, Zambon A, Torchio P, Arico S, Decarli A. Trends of liver cirrhosis mortality in Europe, 1970-1989: age-period-cohort analysis and changing alcohol consumption. *Int J Epidemiol* 1997; 26: 100-9.
57. Leifman H, Romelsjo A. The effect of changes in alcohol consumption on mortality and admissions with alcohol-related diagnoses in Stockholm County. A time series analysis. *Addiction* 1997; 92: 1523-36.
58. Bullock KD, Reed RJ, Grant I. Reduced mortality risk in alcoholics who achieve long-term abstinence. *JAMA* 1992; 267: 668-72.
59. Ratziu V, Bonyhay L, Di Martino V, Charlotte F, Cavallaro L, Sayegh-Tainturier MH, Giral P, Grimaldi A, Opolon P, Poynard T. Survival, liver failure, and hepatocellular carcinoma in obesity-related cryptogenic cirrhosis. *Hepatology* 2002; 35: 1485-93.
60. Niederau C, Fischer R, Purschel A, Stremmel W, Haussinger D, Strohmeyer G. Long-term survival in patients with hereditary hemochromatosis. *Gastroenterology* 1996; 110: 1107-19.
61. Milman N, Pedersen P, a Steig T, Byg KE, Graudal N, Fenger K. Clinically overt hereditary hemochromatosis in Denmark 1948-1985: epidemiology, factors of significance for long-term survival, and causes of death in 179 patients. *Ann Hematol* 2001; 80: 737-44.
62. Imbert-Bismut F, Ratziu V, Pieroni L, Charlotte F, Benhamou Y, Poynard T. Biochemical markers of liver fibrosis in patients with hepatitis C virus infection: a prospective study. *Lancet* 2001; 357; 1069-75.

Achevé d'imprimer par Corlet, Imprimeur, S.A.
14110 Condé-sur-Noireau (France)
N° d'Imprimeur : 60623 - Dépôt légal : octobre 2002

Imprimé en U.E.